Nanotechnology in Food Products

WORKSHOP SUMMARY

Leslie Pray and Ann Yaktine, *Rapporteurs*

Food Forum

Food and Nutrition Board

INSTITUTE OF MEDICINE
OF THE NATIONAL ACADEMIES

THE NATIONAL ACADEMIES PRESS
Washington, D.C.
www.nap.edu

THE NATIONAL ACADEMIES PRESS • 500 Fifth Street, N.W. • Washington, DC 20001

NOTICE: The project that is the subject of this report was approved by the Governing Board of the National Research Council, whose members are drawn from the councils of the National Academy of Sciences, the National Academy of Engineering, and the Institute of Medicine.

This study was supported by Contract Nos. AG-3A94-C-09-0025 (U.S. Department of Agriculture), N01-OD-4-2139 (National Institutes of Health), and HHSF223200811169P (Food and Drug Administration) between the National Academy of Sciences. Additional support came from Abbott Laboratories, Cargill, Coca-Cola Company, ConAgra Foods, General Mills, Kellogg Company, Kraft Foods, Mars, McDonalds, Mead Johnson Nutrition, Monsanto, and PepsiCo. Any opinions, findings, conclusions, or recommendations expressed in this publication are those of the author(s) and do not necessarily reflect the view of the organizations or agencies that provided support for this project.

International Standard Book Number-13: 978-0-309-13772-0
International Standard Book Number-10: 0-309-13772-1

Additional copies of this report are available from the National Academies Press, 500 Fifth Street, N.W., Lockbox 285, Washington, DC 20055; (800) 624-6242 or (202) 334-3313 (in the Washington metropolitan area); Internet, http://www.nap.edu.

For more information about the Institute of Medicine, visit the IOM home page at **www.iom.edu.**

Copyright 2009 by the National Academy of Sciences. All rights reserved.

Printed in the United States of America

The serpent has been a symbol of long life, healing, and knowledge among almost all cultures and religions since the beginning of recorded history. The serpent adopted as a logotype by the Institute of Medicine is a relief carving from ancient Greece, now held by the Staatliche Museen in Berlin.

Suggested citation: IOM (Institute of Medicine). 2009. *Nanotechnology in food products: Workshop Summary*. Washington, DC: The National Academies Press.

*"Knowing is not enough; we must apply.
Willing is not enough; we must do."*
—Goethe

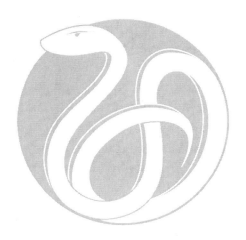

INSTITUTE OF MEDICINE
OF THE NATIONAL ACADEMIES

Advising the Nation. Improving Health.

THE NATIONAL ACADEMIES
Advisers to the Nation on Science, Engineering, and Medicine

The **National Academy of Sciences** is a private, nonprofit, self-perpetuating society of distinguished scholars engaged in scientific and engineering research, dedicated to the furtherance of science and technology and to their use for the general welfare. Upon the authority of the charter granted to it by the Congress in 1863, the Academy has a mandate that requires it to advise the federal government on scientific and technical matters. Dr. Ralph J. Cicerone is president of the National Academy of Sciences.

The **National Academy of Engineering** was established in 1964, under the charter of the National Academy of Sciences, as a parallel organization of outstanding engineers. It is autonomous in its administration and in the selection of its members, sharing with the National Academy of Sciences the responsibility for advising the federal government. The National Academy of Engineering also sponsors engineering programs aimed at meeting national needs, encourages education and research, and recognizes the superior achievements of engineers. Dr. Charles M. Vest is president of the National Academy of Engineering.

The **Institute of Medicine** was established in 1970 by the National Academy of Sciences to secure the services of eminent members of appropriate professions in the examination of policy matters pertaining to the health of the public. The Institute acts under the responsibility given to the National Academy of Sciences by its congressional charter to be an adviser to the federal government and, upon its own initiative, to identify issues of medical care, research, and education. Dr. Harvey V. Fineberg is president of the Institute of Medicine.

The **National Research Council** was organized by the National Academy of Sciences in 1916 to associate the broad community of science and technology with the Academy's purposes of furthering knowledge and advising the federal government. Functioning in accordance with general policies determined by the Academy, the Council has become the principal operating agency of both the National Academy of Sciences and the National Academy of Engineering in providing services to the government, the public, and the scientific and engineering communities. The Council is administered jointly by both Academies and the Institute of Medicine. Dr. Ralph J. Cicerone and Dr. Charles M. Vest are chair and vice chair, respectively, of the National Research Council.

www.national-academies.org

PLANNING COMMITTEE FOR A WORKSHOP ON NANOTECHNOLOGY IN FOOD PRODUCTS: IMPACT ON FOOD SCIENCE, NUTRITION, AND THE CONSUMER[1]

MICHAEL P. DOYLE (*Chair*), University of Georgia, Griffin
JANET BEAUVAIS, Health Canada, Ottawa, Ontario
HONGDA CHEN, U.S. Department of Agriculture, Washington, DC
ERIC DECKER, University of Massachusetts, Amherst
EDWARD GROTH III, Groth Consulting Services, Pelham, NY
DARLENE HARDIE-MUNCY, Cargill Corporation, Wayzata, MN
VAN HUBBARD, National Institutes of Health, Bethesda, MD
DONNA V. PORTER, Library of Congress, Washington, DC
GEORGE PUGH, Coca-Cola Company, Atlanta, GA

Study Staff

ANN YAKTINE, Study Director
GERALDINE KENNEDO, Administrative Assistant

---

[1] Institute of Medicine planning committees are solely responsible for organizing the workshop, identifying topics, and choosing speakers. The responsibility for the published workshop summary rests with the workshop rapporteurs and the institution.

FOOD FORUM[1]

MICHAEL P. DOYLE (*Chair*), University of Georgia, Griffin
MARK ANDON, ConAgra Foods Inc., Omaha, NE
RHONA APPLEBAUM, The Coca-Cola Company, Atlanta, Georgia
SUSAN BORRA, Edelman, Washington, DC
FRANK BUSTA, University of Minnesota, St. Paul
JULIE CASWELL, University of Massachusetts, Amherst
CELESTE A. CLARK, Kellogg Company, Battle Creek, MI
DAVID B. COCKRAM, Abbott Laboratories, Columbus, OH
SUSAN J. CROCKETT, General Mills, Minneapolis, MN
PETER VAN DAEL, Mead Johnson Nutrition, Evansville, IN
ERIC A. DECKER, University of Massachusetts, Amherst
DEBRA DEMUTH, McDonalds Corporation, Oak Brook, IL
SAMUEL GODEFROY, Health Canada, Ottawa, Ontario
NED GROTH III, Groth Consulting Services, Pelham, New York
BRENDA HALBROOK, Department of Agriculture, Washington, DC
DARLENE HARDIE-MUNCY, Cargill, Wayzata, MN
JERRY HJELLE, Monsanto Company, St. Louis, MO
VAN S. HUBBARD, National Institutes of Health, Bethesda, MD
GORDON L. JENSEN, Pennsylvania State University, University Park
CAROL KELLAR, Kraft Foods, Glenview, IL
CHOR-SAN KHOO, Campbell Soup Company, Camden, NJ
JOSEPH A. LEVITT, Hogan & Hartson, L.L.P., Washington DC
DONNA PORTER, Library of Congress, Washington, DC
STEPHEN F. SUNDLOF, Food and Drug Administration, Washington DC
CATHERINE E. WOTEKI, Mars, Incorporated, McLean, VA
DEREK YACH, PepsiCo, Purchase, NY
BARRY L. ZOUMAS, Pennsylvania State University, University Park

Study Staff

ANN YAKTINE, Study Director (through February 2009)
CAITLIN BOON, Study Director
GERALDINE KENNEDO, Administrative Assistant
LINDA D. MEYERS, Director, Food and Nutrition Board

---

[1] Institute of Medicine forums and roundtables do not issue, review, or approve individual documents. The responsibility for the published workshop summary rests with the workshop rapporteurs and the institution.

Reviewers

This report has been reviewed in draft form by individuals chosen for their diverse perspectives and technical expertise, in accordance with procedures approved by the National Research Council's Report Review Committee. The purpose of this independent review is to provide candid and critical comments that will assist the institution in making its published report as sound as possible and to ensure that the report meets institutional standards for objectivity, evidence, and responsiveness to the study charge. The review comments and draft manuscript remain confidential to protect the integrity of the deliberative process. We wish to thank the following individuals for their review of this report:

Eric A. Decker, Department of Food Science, University of Massachusetts

Donna V. Porter, Congressional Research Service, Library of Congress

Patrick J. Stover, Division of Nutritional Sciences, Cornell University

Although the reviewers listed above have provided many constructive comments and suggestions, they were not asked to endorse the final draft of the report before its release. The review of this report was overseen by **Sanford A. Miller,** Joint Institute for Food Safety and Applied Nutrition, University of Maryland. Appointed by the Institute of Medicine, he was responsible for making certain that an independent examination of this report was carried out in accordance with institutional procedures and that all review comments were carefully considered. Responsibility for the final content of this report rests entirely with the authors and the institution.

Contents

Overview

Nanotechnology is giving scientists the means to make and manipulate matter at a size scale never before possible and create novel structures with highly unique properties and wide-ranging applications. Manufacturing industries are actively exploring potential applications of nanotechnology, and many products made with nanoengineered materials are entering the marketplace. In the food industry, scientists are exploring nanotech's potential to encapsulate and deliver nutrients directly into targeted tissues, enhance the flavor and other sensory characteristics of foods, and introduce antibacterial nanostructures into foods, among other applications. The potential benefits are not just in foods themselves but also in the things that "surround" foods, like food packaging, food processing and sensory systems, and basic food and nutrition science research.

However, as with any new technology, along with the intended and ancillary benefits of these applications, there will likely be unanticipated adverse effects. There is still a great deal to learn about the nutritional and safety consequences of introducing nanosized materials into foods and food packaging materials. For example, how do the properties of nanomaterials change when introduced into different types of food matrices or migrate from packaging materials into foods? What happens when nanomaterials interact with a unique biological system such as the human gut? And what is required for evaluating and balancing the potential benefits and risks of introducing nanosized materials into foods and, via those foods, into the human body? Developing nanotechnology into a safe, effective tool for use in food science and technology will require addressing these and other questions. Assuring consumer confidence will be equally important to the success of this new emerging technology.

1

On December 10, 2008, the Institute of Medicine (IOM) held a one-day workshop to further explore the use of nanotechnology in food. Specifically, the workshop was organized around three primary topic areas: (1) the application of nanotechnology to food products ("Session 1"); (2) the safety and efficacy of nanomaterials in food products ("Session 2"); and (3) educating and informing consumers about the applications of nanotechnology to food products ("Session 3"). Ten experts who have been involved in food nanotechnology since its inception and who are recognized as world authorities in the field were invited to give presentations. Each session comprised three or four presentations, followed by open discussion.

This report is a summary of the presentations and discussions that took place during the workshop. The organization of the workshop report parallels the organization of the workshop itself, with the Session 1 presentations and discussions summarized in Chapter 2 ("Application of Nanotechnology to Food Products"); Session 2 presentations and discussions summarized in Chapter 3 ("Safety and Efficacy of Nanomaterials in Food Products"); and Session 3 presentations and discussions summarized in Chapter 4 ("Educating and Informing Consumers About Applications of Nanotechnology to Food Products"). Each chapter begins with an overview of the major issues addressed during that session.

The meeting transcripts and presentations served as the basis for the summary. The agenda for the workshop appears in Appendix A, and Appendix B lists the workshop participants. Appendix C contains the biographical sketches for the presenters, moderators, and panelists. Appendix D lists acronyms and abbreviations used throughout the workshop. The reader should be aware that the material presented here expresses the views and opinions of individuals participating in the workshop either as presenters, panelists or audience members, and not the deliberations or conclusions of a formally constituted IOM committee. The objective of the workshop was not to come to consensus on any single issue. Nor was the goal to comprehensively address all pertinent food safety issues. It was to examine ways that nanotechnology applications in food and nutrients can contribute to the wellbeing of the general public and safety of nanotechnology in food products. These proceedings summarize only the statements of workshop participants and are not intended to be an exhaustive exploration of the subject matter.

Food Forum Chair Michael Doyle opened the meeting with some brief introductory remarks. While there would be some discussion later during the workshop around the lack of consensus regarding a specific definition of nanotechnology (or nanotechnolog*ies*), nanotechnology as a term generally defines objects that fall within the 1 to 100 nanometer (nm) scale, with 1 nm equaling one-billionth of a meter (10^{-9} m), As Doyle put it, nanomaterials are so small, even bacteria would need a microscope to see them! Nano-sized structures can do "incredible" things, Doyle said, when they are applied to foods—they can change the color, smell, or other sensory characteristics, and they can alter the nutritional functionality. Some key questions remain, however, regarding the nutritional and safety consequences of using nanomaterials as food components. The purpose of the workshop, Doyle said, was to discuss the applications of nanotechnology in food, the potential benefits for food safety and nutrition applications, and issues of safety and consumer concerns about the use of nanotechnologies in food.

Doyle acknowledged members of the planning committee, then introduced the first speaker of the day, Rickey Yada, whom Doyle said would be providing an overview of nanotechnology and opportunities for it to be applied in foods, food packaging, and nutrient delivery. A paraphrased summary of Yada's presentation is provided in Chapter 1.

1

Introduction

Rickey Yada opened the meeting with his introductory presentation, *Nanotechnology: A New Frontier in Foods, Food Packaging, and Nutrient Delivery*. Yada provided an overview of the definition(s) and history of nanotechnology, emphasizing that food scientists and technologists have been working with naturally existing nanomaterials and nanoscale phenomona long before modern-day nanotechnology emerged; an overview of the different types of modern-day nanotechnologies being applied in the food industry and how they are being or could be applied; and a summary of key issues that will need to be addressed as the field moves forward. He emphasized the need to fill gaps in understanding the benefits, safety, and environmental consequences of using nanotechnology in food; and the need for transparency and the establishment of public trust. Yada touched on many issues that would be revisited in greater detail or at greater length later during the workshop. A summary of his presentation follows. But first, this chapter begins with a summary of the several major themes that emerged over the course of the day's dialogue.

MAJOR WORKSHOP THEMES

Several major workshop themes emerged over the course of the day, with issues pertaining to each being revisited by multiple speakers and at different times during the open discussions:

Workshop presenters described many potential applications of nanotechnology in foods, food packaging systems, and other areas of food and nutrition science and technology. Some of these applications have already appeared in consumer goods, although most are still in the research and development phase. Rickey Yada, Jose Aguilera, Frans

5

Kampers, and Jochen Weiss each described some of these applications during their presentations. However, as Yada and, later, Martin Philbert, stated, there is a difference between "nano-fact" and "nano-fiction": many of the more "futuristic" applications being touted (not just in food but with nanotechnology in general) may never be realized.

Throughout the day, presenters and other workshop attendees touched upon a wide range of potential benefits of these applications. The potential benefits of food nanotechnology extend across many different areas of food and nutrition science and technology, including basic research (e.g., the use of nanoscale instrumentation to analyze nanoscale food processing phenomena in ways not possible in the past), nutrition (e.g., the use of nanomaterials to encapsulate and deliver nutrients to targeted tissues), food technology (e.g., the use of nanotechnology-based labels on food products as a way to provide consumers with real-time information about the quality of the product), and even medicine (e.g., the use of nanomaterial-based nutrient delivery systems as an interventional health strategy).

Workshop presenters identified several gaps in knowledge about the nutritional and safety consequences of introducing nano-sized structures into foods, and several participants expressed uncertainty about how best to evaluate the potential benefits versus risks of nanotechnology. During their presentations, both Aguilera and Philbert described some of the gaps in knowledge about what happens to nanomaterials when introduced, firstly, into a food matrix and, secondly, into the human body. As Philbert elaborated, along with intended (and ancillary) benefits, there will likely be unintended adverse effects. For example, there may be unanticipated risks associated not so much with the actual nanomaterials but with some of the other, non-nano substances used to ensure that the nanomaterials behave in their intended manner. So far, no real safety issues or incidents have been identified. But as the field moves forward, as both Philbert and Jean Halloran emphasized, weighing the potential benefits against potential risks will be crucial to developing food nanotechnology into a safe and effective tool. However, as evident by discussion at the end of Sessions 2 and 3 (and as summarized in Chapters 3 and 4), there are many uncertainties around both how the benefits and risks can and should be measured and what specific regulatory measures can and should serve as a framework for evaluation.

There was considerable discussion around the regulatory measures already in place for examining the benefit-risk balance of nanotechology applications in food and the likely need for more complete guidance in the future. During her presentation, Laura Tarantino argued that statutory authorities already provide the U.S. Food and Drug Administration (FDA) with the necessary tools for evaluating and regulating the safety of nanomaterials with novel properties and that the FDA's existing procedures and systems are adequate for evaluating and regulating nanotechnology in food. Tarantino encouraged early and frequent consultation with the FDA so that manufacturers can get a sense of what will be expected of them when their product(s) are ready for review. Fred Degnan agreed with Tarantino about FDA's existing statutory authorities but emphasized the necessity of having at least some sort of written guidance available to industry, even if that guidance is only preliminary and tentative. There was considerable discussion at the end of Sessions 2 and 3 about the timeline and direction of next steps and future options for the FDA and other regulatory agencies.

While many workshop participants agreed that engaging the public is necessary in order to build understanding and ultimately acceptance of this emerging technology, there are still some unanswered questions about how best to proceed. As presenter Julia Moore elaborated, public opinion of nanotechnology is "up for grabs," with very few people knowing anything at all about the use of nanotechnology in food. Now is the time to act, she said. But, as with many of the other issues up for discussion during the workshop, there is uncertainty about how to proceed. For example, while commending presenter Carl Batt for his group's nanotechnology public education efforts, Halloran also questioned whether education necessarily translates into acceptance. As another example, when asked whether there are particular types of nanomaterials or nanotechnology applications that consumers would be more willing to accept in foods, Halloran remarked that the issue is not whether consumers are for or against nanotechnology, rather whether or not nanotechnology provides actual benefits to consumers and is safe. There was considerable discussion at the end of Session 3 on this topic, with participants commenting on consumer choice and decision making (e.g., how consumers perceive benefit and risk), use of the word nanotechnology (e.g., compared to what some participants argued was the more accurate "nanotechnologies"), lessons to be learned from the biotechnology experience, and other related issues.

Again, the purpose of the workshop was neither to reach consensus on any single issue nor come to any conclusions about specific next steps. In fact, an overarching theme of the workshop presentations and discussion was the uncertainty that still exists regarding how best to

move forward on several scientific (e.g., how to evaluate both the benefits and risks of adding synthetic nanomaterials to foods) and societal
(e.g., how to engage the public) fronts.

NANOTECHNOLOGY: A NEW FRONTIER IN FOODS, FOOD PACKAGING, AND NUTRIENT DELIVERY[1]

Presenter: Rickey Yada[2]

Yada began by remarking that nanotechnology holds forth much
promise as a means of providing novel solutions to many of the greatest
problems facing the world today, from energy production (i.e., finding
new ways to produce plentiful, low-cost energy) to food and clean water
shortages. As just one example, he identified water shortage as one of
Canada's biggest problems, with Alberta utilizing a tremendous amount
of non-reusable water for oil recovery; nanotechnology may provide a
means to reuse that water.

The Definition(s) and History of Nanotechnology

Before describing some of the details of potential applications of
nanotechnology in food, Yada talked about the definition(s) and history
of nanotechnology. First, what is nanotechnology? There are several
definitions:

From the National Cancer Institute website[3]: "Technology development at the atomic, molecular, or macromolecular range of approximately 1–100 nanometers to create and use structures, devices, and systems that have novel properties."

Also from the National Cancer Institute website[4]: "Technology on
the nanometer scale. The *original* definition is technology that is built
from single atoms and which depends on individual atoms for function.

---

[1] This section is a paraphrased summary of Rickey Yada's introductory presentation.
[2] Rickey Yada, PhD, is a Professor of Food Science and a Canada Research Chair in
Food Protein Structure at the University of Guelph, Ontario.
[3] Available online at http://plan2005.cancer.gov/glossary.html. Accessed January 19,
2009.
[4] Available online at http://www.ccrnp.ncifcrf.gov/~toms/glossary.html. Accessed January 19, 2009.

An example is an enzyme. If you mutate the enzyme's gene, the modified enzyme may or may not function. In contrast, if you remove a few atoms from a hammer, it still will work just as well. This is an important distinction that has generally been lost as the hype about nanotechnology and it is used as a buzzword for 'small' instead of a distinctly different technology. Fortunately real nanotechnologies are in the works...."

From the European Union–funded NanoHand project website[5]: "Nanotechnology comprises the emerging application of Nanoscience. Nanoscience is dealing with functional systems either based on the use of sub-units with specific size-dependent properties or of individual or combined functionalized sub-units."

From the National Nanotechnology Initiative (NNI): The NNI considers something "nanotechnology" only when nanotechnology tools and concepts are used to study biology; biological molecules are engineered to have functions very different from those they have in nature; and manipulation of biological systems is done by methods more precise than can be done by using molecular biological, synthetic chemical, or biochemical approaches that have been used for years in the biology research community.

Elsewhere, nanotechnology is often generally defined as any technology dealing with objects within the 1–100 nm range. But without having a sense of what kind of objects are 1–100 nm long, many people have a difficult time relating to this length scale. Yada considered the fourth definition above to be the "most pragmatic." Even more useful, he said, is defining nanotechnology and nanoscience by using a visual display of nanosized natural and manufactured objects, so that consumers and the public can see descriptive objects in relationship to the length scale (see Figure 1-1).

[5] Available online at http://www.nanohand.eu/index.php?page=114&include_link=glossary#N. Accessed January 19, 2009.

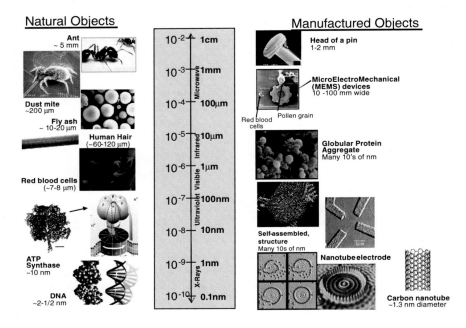

FIGURE 1-1 A visual display of natural and manufactured objects that fall in the "nano" (<100 nm) and "micro" (>100 nm) size ranges. Image courtesy of Jochen Weiss and the U.S. Department of Energy.[6]

Yada emphasized that nanotechnology is not a new field. The only truly new thing about nanotechnology, he said, is that "we have been able to capture it under a rubric called nanotechnology." Scientists have been studying "nanoscience" phenomena for more than a century. Louis Pasteur's work with spoilage bacteria (1866), Watson and Crick's discovery of the structure of DNA (1953), can be considered nanoscience as well as Richard Smalley's research on buckyballs (1996) and, in fact, each represent major milestones in the "science of small."

---

[6] This image is a slight modification of "The Scale of Things" chart developed by the Office of Basic Energy Sciences, Office of Science, U.S. Department of Energy. The original can be viewed online at http://www.er.doe.gov/bes/scale_of_things.html.

Pasteur's work with spoilage bacteria, measurable on the micrometer (μm) scale (1 μm = 1000 nanometers), led to a revolution in food processing and the development of safer, better quality foods.

Getting smaller, Watson and Crick's discovery of the structure of DNA (a molecule of DNA is about 2.5 nm wide) led to a biotechnology revolution and the development of better biomedical treatments and agricultural production and processes.

Getting even smaller, Smalley's research with buckyballs, which fall within the Å range (10 Å = 1 nm), marked the beginning of the current era of nanoscale science and technology and its unprecedented impacts across broad sectors of society.

Yada noted that Switzerland was the first country to invest heavily in modern nanoscience, in the mid-1990s, with Canada and other countries following suit.

Much of the recent interest in nanoscience has been driven by the development of instrumentation and the availability of tools that allow scientists to see things that they were unable to see in the past. Yada noted that when he was an undergraduate, the concept of "parts per million," or ppm, was a "sort of wonderment." Now, scientists talk in terms that exceed parts per trillion, because there is instrumentation that allows them to see those parts (e.g., transmission electron and atomic force microscopy, scanning tunneling X-ray). This is not surprising, Yada noted, since research often follows developments in technology. For example, most food science departments originated as dairy departments but, as processing and other techniques developed, those dairy departments transitioned into "food science" departments.

Today, much of the fascination with nanotechnology is in the area of drug delivery, with many products in phase I, II, or III clinical trial. Examples of nano-sized commercial products include paliperidone palmitate nanocrystals for the treatment of schizophrenia and paclitaxel nanoparticles for the treatment of tumors. Yada mentioned how people have imagined the notion of targeted drug delivery extending to implantable sensors and surgical robots. He quoted Helen Thomson, the author of a Fall 2008 article on nanotechnology in *Trek*, a magazine published by the University of British Columbia (UBC) Office of Alumni Affairs[7]: "Implantable sensors could allow for continuous and detailed health monitoring so illness might be detected and treated sooner. Surgical

---

[7] H Thomson. 2008. Is nanotechnology the next big thing or the next big nightmare? *Trek* Fall:15-17.

robots introduced into living tissue could excise harmful cells and repair damaged ones." But are implantable sensors and surgical robots reality ("nano-fact'), or are they Jules Verne–style science fiction ("nano-fiction")? Yada also referred to the movie *Fantastic Voyage* (a 1966 film), where a tiny submarine is injected into a person so that the crew of the submarine could perform surgery, and wondered if nanotechnology might be "where science fiction becomes reality."

Applications of Nanotechnology in the Food Industry

Food technology experts have identified four major types of applications of nanotechnology in the food industry: (1) agriculture, (2) food processing, (3) food packaging, and (4) supplements (see Table 1-1). But this categorization, Yada explained, is somewhat arbitrary and based on ease of compartmentalization. The really interesting nanoscience, he said, is happening where these different application areas intersect. Solving these more interesting problems will require coordinated, interdisciplinary efforts among food engineers, food chemists, food microbiologists, and others. For example, taking their cues from nanomedicine, food scientists have adopted the concept of targeted drug delivery and are actively researching targeted nutrient delivery intervention strategies that could help people maintain their health. Yada commented on how this bridging of the food-medicine gap has created a common theme and led to a greater dialogue between food and nutrient scientists. He described how the Food Science department at the University of Guelph is separated from the Nutritional Science department by a delivery alleyway and that there had been very little interaction between the two departments for many years. This was true despite the fact that both departments deal with food; the only difference between them is that Food Science focuses on how that food is processed and preserved, Nutritional Science on the nutritional consequences of that food once it is inside the human body. But over the past five years or so, the two departments have begun consolidating their expertise in efforts to develop new nutrient delivery systems. While few, if any, food–related commercial applications for controlled release are available, there are a limited number of other types of nano-sized commercial products available (e.g., nanoceutials, Nutrition-be-nanotech, Aquanova) that were derived from this type of convergence of expertise (i.e., not necessarily at the University of Guelph but generally).

TABLE 1-1 Overview of the Wide-Ranging Potential Applications of Nanotechnology Being Researched, Tested, and in Some Cases Already Applied in the Food Industry

Agriculture	Food Processing	Food Packaging	Supplements
Nanotechnology-enabled single molecule detection for determining enzyme/substrate interactions	Nanocapsules for improving bioavailability of neutraceuticals in standard ingredients such as cooking oils	Fluorescent nanoparticles with attached antibodies for detecting chemicals or foodborne pathogens	Nanosize powders for increasing absorption of nutrients
Nanopsules for delivery of pesticides, fertilizers, and other agrichemicals more efficiently	Nanoencapsulated flavor enhancers	Biodegradable nanosensors for temperature, moisture, and time monitoring	Cellulose nanocrystal composites as drug carriers
Nanotechnology-enabled delivery of growth hormones in a controlled fashion	Nanotubes and nanoparticles as gelation and viscosifying agents	Nanoclays and nano-films as barrier materials to prevent spoilage and oxygen absorption	Nanocochleates (coiled nanoparticles) for more efficient nutrient delivery to cells without affecting color or taste of food
Nanosensors for monitoring soil conditions and crop growth	Nanocapsule infusions of plant-based steroids as a replacement for meat cholesterol	Electrochemical nanosensors for detecting ethylene	Vitamin sprays that disperse nanodroplets with better absorption
Nanochips for identity preservation and tracking	Nanoparticles that selectively bind and remove chemicals or pathogens from food	Nanoparticle-containing antimicrobial and antifungal surface coatings	

Continued

TABLE 1-1 Continued

Nanosensors for detecting animal and plant pathogens	Nanoemulsions and nanoparticles for better availability and dispersion of nutrients	Lighter, stronger, and more heat-resistant films made of silicate nanoparticles
Nanocapsules for vaccine delivery		Nanotechnology-enabled modified permeation behavior of foils
Nanoparticles for NDA delivery to plants (targeted genetic engineering)		

NOTE: The table is adapted from a figure that both Yada and Philbert showed during their presentations; the source of the original figure is *Nanowerk*. *Nanowerk* is an online nanotechnology and nanoscience information portal; the original figure can be viewed online at http://www.nanowerk.com/spotlight/spotid=1846.php.
SOURCE: Reprinted, with permission, from *Nanowerk*.

Yada highlighted several additional potential applications of food nanotechnology:

1. *Improved delivery of micronutrients and bioactive food components*. He identified four major sets of challenges associated with nutrient delivery: (1) stability (i.e., against heat, pH, and oxidation during food processing), (2) taste and color (i.e., avoiding unpleasant tastes or colors), (3) safety, and (4) bioavailability. Nanotechnology could be used to address each of these. With taste, for example, while people are willing to withstand horrible tasting cough medicines, knowing that the medicines have some therapeutic value, the same is not true of foods. Moreover, consumers are becoming more discerning, wanting more palatable foods than in the past.

2. *Controlled release* (i.e., the controlled release of bioactive compounds, such as omega-3 fatty acids). Just as in medicine, where the aim is to eliminate the potential of under- or over-dosing, the main goal of controlled release of bioactive compounds is to avoid cyclical actions and possible side effects. This has important applications for foods designed for people with diabetes, for example, where it would be desirable to maintain a steady state of glucose release.

3. *Product traceability.* As the recent melamine threat demonstrated, the ability to trace contaminants back to their source is an important component of food safety. Yada pointed to Stephen D. Nightingale's presentation at the 2008 Institute of Food Technologists (IFT) International Food Nanoscience Conference as a source of information on this topic.

4. *Food safety intervention.* While Yada did not elaborate on this potential application, he showed a slide citing R.A. Latour's work on the use of adhesin-specific nanoparticles for the re-removal of pathogenic bacteria from poultry. He mentioned that Frans Kampers would be speaking more on this topic.

5. *The detection of zoonotic diseases.* Zoonotic diseases are a growing problem, and there are many examples of nanotechnology being applied toward prion detection in particular, as well as other food-borne toxins.

6. *The development of new food packaging materials, including nanocomposite polymer films.* Yada referred to the development of "intelligent packaging that allows us to not only prevent some contamination from occurring or prevent its proliferation but also detects other compounds." The classic example of this type of application, he said, is packaging that controls over-ripening and keeps bananas green or yellow for longer. "We've made some developments there," he said. Other improvements being sought include packaging with better oxygen and water vapor transmission barrier properties, stronger mechanical properties, and improved thermal stability.

He then briefly described some fabrication approaches being used to construct novel nano-sized food structures and explained how these nano-scale structures add nutritional functionality and value to food. He noted that many of these fabrication approaches are being studied at the U.S. Department of Agriculture (USDA) Cooperative State Research,

Education, and Extension Service (CSREES) (which operates in partnership with the 16 other federal agencies that comprise the National Nanotechnology Initiative [NNI]):

- The use of *nano-scale agricultural foodstocks* to develop new materials with new functionalities. Yada used corn zein as an example of a raw agricultural material being studied for its potential to serve as a nano-size building block of new food materials with added value.
- The use of *milk protein nanotubes* to add functionality. Yada said that "no longer will milk be that substance that we drink three times a day in a glass." Milk is now being fractionated so that some of those fractionated components (e.g., milk protein nanotubes, casein micelles) can be used for other purposes, for example to deliver nutraceuticals.[8]
- The use of *nanostructured fluids* to develop new functionalities that have not existed in the past.
- The use of *nanoemulsions* (i.e., nanostructured emulsions) to serve as a platform for nutrient delivery, for example by encapsulating iron in a food product (e.g., rice) in a way that is palatable to consumers. Normally, iron forms a brown solution, which most people would find unpalatable. But nanoemulsion technology provides a way to coat rice with iron in such a way that the iron is transparent to the eye. Yada identified this technology as one that "may allow us to feed portions of the world that are deficient in certain minerals and vitamins." Yada also pointed to the use of sugar beet pectin as a component in the microencapsulation of lipophilic food ingredients (i.e., molecules and vitamins),[9] which also serves as another example of how naturally existing nano-sized agricultural foodstocks can be used in nanotechnology.

Yada mentioned the use of solid lipid nanoparticles (SLNs) as another platform of delivery and cited Dérick Rousseau's presentation at the 2008 IFT International Food Nanoscience Conference. SLNs are

---

[8] E.g., see E Semo, E Kesselman, D Danino, and YD Livney. 2007. Casein micelle as a natural nano-capsular vehicle for nutraceuticals. *Food Hydrocolloids* 21:936-942.

[9] E.g., see S Drusch. 2007. Sugar beet pectin: A novel emulsifying wall component for microencapsulation of lipophilic food ingredients by spray-drying. *Food Hydrocolloids* 2:1223-1228.

nanoparticles made from solid lipids by high pressure homogenization. Added ingredients can be incorporated into the lipid matrix. Yada commented that Jochen Weiss would be describing SLNs in more detail later during this workshop see Chapter 2.

Issues

"Nanotechnology has been called a molecular revolution—innovation so profound it will allow us to rebuild our world molecule by molecule. The unprecedented benefits of such control over matter have the potential to permeate every aspect of our lives. But so do the risks."
                                                —Hilary Thomson, 2008[10]

Yada began his discussion of the societal implications of nanotechnology with this quote from Thomson. He noted that while studying and developing these various applications of nanotechnology in food, there are also several issues about the consequences of nanotechnology that will need to be addressed in order to alleviate consumer concerns. For example, can nanoparticles pass the blood-brain barrier, and is this passage harmful? Does modification of natural nanoparticles in food pose a risk? What is the effect of the food matrix? What safety data will be required by global food authorities? Yada listed five sets of issues that must be addressed:

1. *Transparency.* Many analogies have been drawn between nanotechnology and genetically modified organisms (GMOs), with many consumers worried about whether nanotechnology will be deemed harmful 5 or 10 years in the future, even if and when the science is deemed safe today. Yada described the issue as a "philosophical debate." There is, however, an important difference between GMO and nanotechnology: There were regulations in place for the monitoring and regulation of GM foods (i.e., the same regulations that had been used to monitor and regulate foods developed through traditional breeding). There are important unanswered questions about whether the risk assessment and management systems traditionally used for chemical and microbial contamination are going to be adopted or if new

---

[10] H Thomson. 2008. Is nanotechnology the next big thing or the next big nightmare? *Trek* Fall:15-17.

ones are going to be developed. Either way, he said, "One has to remember that we probably have to adopt the same kind of framework and concerns that we would for anything else and not become alarmists in this new technology." Many of the regulatory issues are the same as they are for any other new technology (e.g., low acceptance of risk, low profit margin, type of safety data required by food authorities globally).

2. *Education.* Public education, especially among children, needs to improve with respect to understanding nanotechnology (as well as other technologies). Yada quoted Neal Lane, former science advisor to President Clinton: "In the beginning, an explicit aim of the U.S. National Nanotechnology Intitiative (NNI) ... was to excite young girls and boys about science, particularly the physical sciences and engineering. The intent was to reach millions of children using the wonders of nanotechnology to encourage them to study science and to equip them to compete successfully at the cutting-edge of a globalized economy." The question is: How do we teach children to be critical of the information that is so readily available right at their fingertips? Yada mentioned just having finished teaching a course where he had students believing that information available on the Internet is true, simply by virtue of it's being on the Internet, in much the same way that past generations believed that if something was reported in the newspaper, it must be true.

3. *Benefits.* What are the societal impacts of nanotechnology? Who will benefit, and who will pay? Yada referred to a 2003 report on the societal implications of nanotechnology published by the Nanoscale Science, Engineering and Technology (NSET) Subcommittee of the National Science and Technology Council's Committee on Technology: www.nano.gov/nni_societal_ implications.pdf. For more information on the benefits of nanotechnology, Yada also referenced a more recent Project on Emerging Nanotechnologies newsletter dedicated to the topic of nanotechnology (*Nanotechnology: Energizing the Future*): www.nanotechproject.org/publications/archive/nanotechnology_ energizing_future/. The newsletter continues and updates a discussion on nanotechnology that took place at a 2006 meeting co-sponsored by the Project on Emerging Nanotechnologies, National Institutes of Health, and the National Science Foundation (NSF).

4. *Consumer safety.* Yada referenced the World Nanofood Report (http://www.fiweekly.com/WNR1108.pdf) and a Canadian Academies report, Small is Different: A Science Perspective on the Regulatory Challenges of the Nanoscale (http://www.science advice.ca/documents/(2008_07_10)_Report_on_Nanotechnology .pdf), both of which address safety and regulatory issues surrounding the use of nanotechnology in food. The latter report addresses the issue of unknown potential hazards.

5. *Environmental impact.* Yada quoted the Trek magazine article on nanotechnology again: "[UBC assistant professor Milind] Kandlikar says ... scientists just don't know what properties—shape, size, chemical composition or coatings—might make nanoparticles and nanowaste hazardous." He referred workshop participants to a website describing activities of a recently developed center, jointly run by Duke University and University of California, Los Angeles, and funded by NSF and the U.S. Environmental Protection Agency (EPA), for examining the potential hazards of nanomaterials: www.cenonline.org.

In conclusion, Yada again quoted the *Trek* magazine article: "Nanotechnology could be the first technology developed with sensitivity to ethical, environmental and social issues. If we fearlessly and responsibly examine all aspects of the technology today, we can anticipate our tomorrow will be enriched with benefits." He said that the benefits of nanotechnology are enormous, with many potential and exciting products on the market. But so too are the challenges. There are major gaps in our understanding of the health, safety, environmental, and societal impacts of nanotechnology. Filling these gaps will be critically important to the long-term success of nanotechnology.

Finally, Yada reemphasized that food nanoscience represents a university research culture shift and that filling these gaps will require a multidisciplinary approach, and he stressed the importance of building public trust in the science and industry of nanotechnology. Controversial issues surrounding nanotechnology have already sparked public interest in the field. Establishing public trust and developing and maintaining the credibility of nanoscience will require a coherent and rational approach on behalf of the scientific enterprise, careful planning and strategic coordination, and the bringing together of the necessary multidisciplinary team with a networking mindset.

2

Application of Nanotechnology to Food Products

This chapter summarizes the presentations and discussions of the first session of the workshop. All three presentations revolved around the question: How can nanotechnology be applied in the food industry? The first presenter, José Miguel Aguilera of Universidad Católica de Chile, Santiago, discussed how nanotechnology will provide new ways of controlling and structuring foods with greater functionality and value. But first, he talked about how "nano" has, in fact, been part of food processing for centuries, since many food structures naturally exist at the nano-scale. Until very recently, however, most of what has been done with nano-sized food materials has occurred in a largely uncontrolled way, and there is still a lot to be learned about the natural nano-structure of foods (e.g., how foods are constructed and how they break down during digestion). Until and unless these gaps in knowledge are filled, scientists could miss opportunities to apply some of the new nanotechnologies being developed. The second presenter, Frans Kampers of Wageningen UR, Wageningen, The Netherlands, argued that nanotechnology holds forth tremendous promise to provide benefits not just within food products but also around food products. In other words, not only can nanotechnology be used to structure new types of food ingredients, it can also be used to build new types of food packages, food quality detection tools, and other types of measurement and detection systems. He described some of the work that Wageningen UR scientists and others are doing in the areas of volatile sensing, microorganism detection, and food labeling. Kampers stated that these types of applications are arguably noncontroversial, or at least less controversial than some of the food ingredient applications of nanotechnology, and as such could serve as a "stepping stone for the general public to appreciate what nanotechnologies can offer to the food industry and where benefits for consumers can be derived from these technologies."

The third presenter, Jochen Weiss of the University of Massachusetts, Amherst, provided an overview of how nanotechnologies are being developed to add novel functionalities to food products. He described several different nanomaterials currently being explored for their potential applications in food products, including microemulsions, liposomes, solid lipid nanoparticles (SLNs), and nanofibers. He also described some of the research that he and his colleagues have been conducting with each of these types of materials, emphasizing the variety of ways one can build nanostructured materials with potent, long-lasting antimicrobial capacities. In fact, scientists are beginning to construct all sorts of different types of microscopic structures with varying functionalities (not just antimicrobial capacities) using nanomaterials as their building blocks. What scientists don't fully understand yet, however, is how these structures will function once inside actual food systems.

The session ended with a 20-minute question and answer period, with most of the discussion revolving around the commercial availability of these various applications and products, the definition and history of nanotechnology, and regulatory uncertainty. The last topic—regulatory uncertainty—would re-emerge in later sessions as a major overarching theme of the workshop dialogue. There was also some discussion on the issue of palatability and nutrient delivery and whether nanotechnology offers any solutions.

APPLICATIONS OF NANOSCIENCES TO NUTRIENTS AND FOODS[1]

Presenter: José Miguel Aguilera[2]

Aguilera began with some introductory remarks about his work as a food microstructure engineer and how, in the past, the focus of his research was on larger food structures (i.e., "micron-size"). Now, he is trying to extrapolate what he has learned about the structure of foods at that micro-level to a smaller scale. He provided a brief outline of his presentation, with a reminder that "we already have a lot of nanotech in

---

[1] This section is a paraphrased summary of Jose Miguel Aguilera's presentation.
[2] José Miguel Aguilera, PhD, is a Professor in the Department of Chemical and Bioprocess Engineering, Universidad Católica de Chile, Santiago, Chile.

our foods." The focus of his talk, he said, would be on how foods are structured today, how they could be structured in the future by reducing the scale of intervention, and the implications of the latter for adding unique value to foods with respect to nutrition/health and gastronomy/pleasure. The smallest food microstructure that can be controlled with current processing technologies is probably only about 5–10 μm, which is about 100 times larger than the upper limit of nanotechnology. So there is a big gap between what current technologies can do and the promise that nanotechnology holds forth.

Introduction: The Food Industry and the Role of Nanosciences

The food industry is the largest manufacturing sector in the world, with an annual turnover approximating US $4 trillion. But it presents a very different innovation scenario than the chemical and pharma industries do, and introducing new processing technologies (e.g., high hydrostatic pressure [HHP] technology, -ohmic heating, irradiation) has been challenging. Globally, a large proportion of foods are consumed after only minimal processing (e.g., fresh fruits, vegetables, nuts, some cereals) and with high post-harvest losses (particularly with fruits and vegetables). In most places worldwide, particularly in urban centers, food is abundant and relatively cheap. Moreover, except for large multinationals, most food companies are relatively low-tech, small/medium enterprises (SMEs) where traditional technologies are geared to local tastes and traditions.

The Two Axes of Today's Food Industry

Aguilera described two axes, or dimensions, of the food industry of today and the food industry of the future (see Figure 2-1):

1. The "food chain" axis, which extends from production to packaging and distribution (and includes raw materials, processing, and all of the various environmental and technological factors that contribute).
2. The "consumer" axis, which extends from the brain to the mouth on one end (and includes things like food perception and

pleasure) and from the mouth to the body on the other end (affecting things like bioavailability of nutrients, weight control, and satiety).

He remarked that the second axis has been part of the food industry for only the last 10–15 years, and it will probably play an even more prominent role in the future. Foods of the future will be built to meet consumer demands and desires around food perception, sensations of wellness and pleasure, texture and flavor, gut health, nutrient bioavailability, vitality, etc.

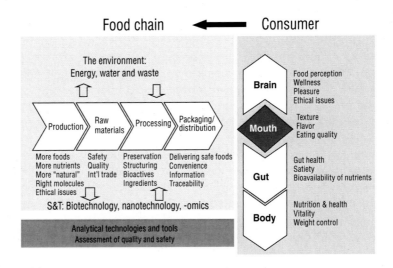

FIGURE 2-1 The two dimensions, or axes, of the food industry of the future: the "food chain" axis and the "consumer" axis. Image courtesy of José Miguel Aguilera.

Where Is the Nano in Foods?

Aguilera remarked that "nano" must exist naturally in food since even in natural foods (e.g., fresh fruits) structural components are built from molecules and, during digestion, break down into molecules. These molecules form ordered structures like cells, fibers, gels, emulsions, foams, and liquids, which give foods their various properties (e.g., texture, flavor, shelf-life, nutritional value). Aguilera showed a variation of the "Scale of Objects" image that Yada showed during his presentation of the micro- vs. nano-scale worlds (see Figure 2-2 and Figure 1-1 for comparison), with pictures and illustrations of "things natural" vs. "things in foods" along a size scale, ranging from 0.1 nm to 1 cm. He agreed with Yada that it is a good visual to present to people as a way of explaining the sizes involved with the "microworld" ["microstructure"] versus the "nanoworld" ["nanotechnology"]. Food microstructures include things like plant cells, starch granules, meat fibers, and chloroplasts. Food nanostructures include things like crystalline blocklets of amylopectin molecules (which serve as building blocks for starch granules) and clusters of chlorophyll molecules embedded in lipid bilayers (which serve as building blocks for chloroplasts).

Aguilera identified the cow udder as the most interesting "natural" microdevice (i.e., device for producing micro-sized food ingredients). He explained how a cow udder cell produces casein micelles and fat globules, both key ingredients of milk, with casein micelles ranging in size from 300–400 nm and fat globules ranging in size from 100 nm to 20 μm. Fat globule membranes have a thickness of 4–25 nm. All structured dairy products (e.g., butter, whipped cream, ice cream, milk, cheese, yogurt) are composed of these two ingredients plus an even smaller ingredient, the whey proteins, which ranges in size from 0.001– 0.01 μm. So, in fact, dairy technology is not just a microtechnology but also a nanotechnology, and it has existed for a long time. The dairy industry utilizes these three basic micro- and nano-sized structures to build all sorts of emulsions (butter), foams (ice cream and whipped cream), complex liquids (milk), plastic solids (cheese), and gel networks (yogurt).[3] But much of what has been done in the past with natural micro- and nano-sized structures, not just in the dairy industry but the food industry in general, has been largely uncontrolled. The first comprehensive scientific perspective on a micro-structural view of food was not published until as recently as 1987.

---

[3] See JM Aguilera and DW Stanley. 1999. *Microstructural Principles of Food Processing and Engineering*, 2nd Edition. Heidelberg, Germany: Springer.

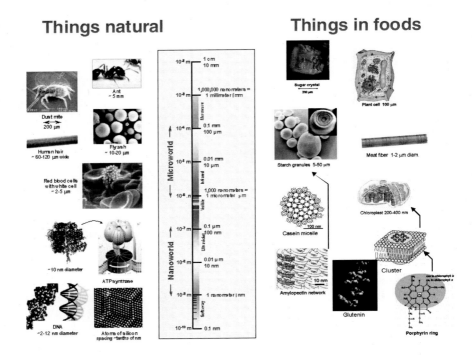

FIGURE 2-2 Similar to the image that Yada showed (see Figure 1-1), this image more clearly represents the difference in scale between nano-sized vs. micro-sized materials and structures *in foods*. Image courtesy of José Miguel Aguilera and the U.S. Department of Energy.[4]

The Scales of Food: Length and Time

Aguilera showed a graph illustrating the range of the length scales of food elements that already exist (either in nature or as a result of processing), emphasizing again that in fact many elements that play very important structural roles in foods that we already eat exist on the nano-scale (see Figure 2-3). We don't notice them because not only are they invisible to the naked eye (most things smaller than about 80 μm cannot be seen by the human eye), they are imperceptible by taste as well (most

---

[4] This image is a modification of "The Scale of Things" chart developed by the Office of Basic Energy Sciences, Office of Science, U.S. Department of Energy. The original can be viewed online at http://www.er.doe.gov/bes/scale_of_things.html.

things smaller than about 40 μm cannot be sensed in the mouth). In fact, some of food's most important raw materials—proteins, starches, and fats—undergo structural changes at the nanometer and micrometer scales during normal food processing (see Figure 2-4):

1. Proteins: Food proteins (e.g., native beta-lactoglobulin, which is about 3.6 nm in length) can undergo denaturation (via pressure, heat, pH, etc.) and the denatured components reassemble to form larger structures, like fibrils or aggregates, which in turn can be assembled to form even larger gel networks (e.g., yogurt). Protein-polysaccharide mixed solutions can spontaneously separate into a phase with nano- or micro-sized droplets dispersed in a continuous phase.

2. Starch: Starch granules expand when heated and hydrated releasing biopolymers that can be recrystallized into nano-sized structures (e.g., recrystallized amylose regions may be about 10–20 nm); dextrins and other degradation products of extrusion can be used to encapsulate bioactive substances in micro-regions, etc.

3. Fats: While many people think of fats as being homogeneous liquids or solids, in fact some fats have a lot of structure. Monoglycerides, for example, can self-assemble into many morphologies at the nanoscale level, and hierarchically structured into tryglicerides can be crystallites (10–100 nm), followed by arrangment into large clusters, then flocs, and finally, fat crystal networks. Fat crystal networks give foods spreadability, texture, and other similar properties.

Aguilera emphasized that all foods, at one stage or another, become dispersions of these multiple interacting components not only with each other but also with water and air. For example, proteins interact with polysaccharides to form mixed polysaccharide gels, starches and proteins interact to form starch-protein complexes, and emulsions and food foams have interfaces that are stabilized by small molecules (surfactants), biopolymers or even small particles.

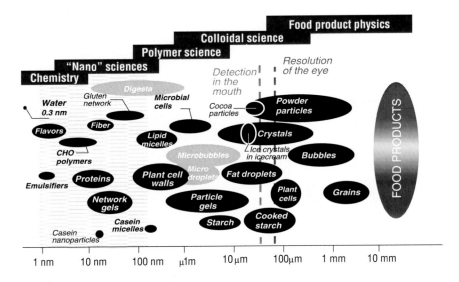

FIGURE 2-3 The length scales of food elements that already exist. Structures to the left of the right dotted line ("Resolution of the eye") are invisible to the naked eye, and structures to the left of the left dotted line ("Detection in the mouth") are imperceptible to taste. Image courtesy of José Miguel Aguilera.

Length is just one scale of measurement for food. Another is time. In order to interact, different components of a food structure must come into position at the right time. The structuring of a foam for example, requires that certain structural components and processes happen not only at specific length scales but also within specific time scales. The beginning of foam formation occurs at the nm-length scale within milliseconds (e.g., adsorption of emulsifier molecules at the air-water interface), whereas later phases of the process occur at larger length scales and longer time scales (e.g., drainage of liquid lamellae occurs at the μm-length scale and within minutes).

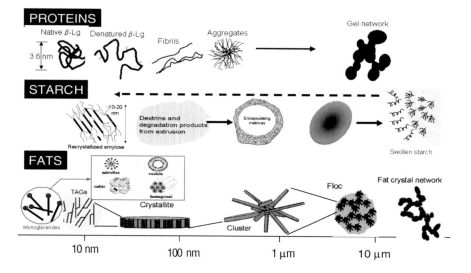

FIGURE 2-4 A schematic of the structural changes that proteins, starch, and fats naturally undergo during normal food processing. Many of these changes occur at the nano-size scale. Image courtesy of José Miguel Aguilera.

How Are Foods Structured Today, and How Should They Be Structured?

Today, foods are structured using a formulation, or recipe, with structure formation (i.e., biopolymer transformation, phase creation, reactions) and stabilization (i.e., vitrification, crystallization, network formation) occurring at the same time. The end result is a metastable structure. In the future, with nanotechnology, foods will be structured from the bottom up. Rather than using a recipe, food structure engineers will use molecules as their starting material, modifying those molecules and building interactions in order to get the desired properties. The process will be more akin to engineering design than recipe-reading, much like how computers and cars are assembled. By building foods from the molecule up, rather than relying on a coupled structure-formation-structure stabilization process, food engineers will utilize an uncoupled "matrix precursors/structural elements" paradigm. That is, microstructural elements will be engineered separately and then dispersed into a matrix precursor, which will have been developed independently. The end product will be a more functional product. As Aguilera said, "the beauty that I see in going down[ward] on the size scale is that we can control and really design and assemble new foods."

Also in the future, not only will food structural engineers be following this architecture-like paradigm, they will be utilizing new tools. Right now, traditional food processing relies on equipment that is capable of intervening at only the microscale (i.e., 10 μm–1 mm), not nanoscale (with some exceptions). Even then, it's like "hammering a nail with a bulldozer," Aguilera said. Emulsification, for example, involves manipulating structural elements that are about 10 μm in length, using a device with an opening of 1 mm—that's two full orders of magnitude difference. As another example, shaping (molding), involves manipulating structural elements that are about 20–30 μm in lengthsize (e.g., bubbles), using a device with an opening devices of 10 cm—that's four orders of magnitude difference. In the future, the scale of intervention will be reduced to the size of the elements being manipulated.

Reducing the Scale of Food Design: Four Examples

Aguilera gave four examples of reduced scale food design, or "controlled structuring" (in each case, the device/method that enables controlled structuring is italicized). The descriptions below accompany the images in Figure 2-5:

1. Architectures of foams made in a 250 μm coaxial *capillary tube* by varying the ratio of gas/liquid flow rates.[5] Here, a microfluidic device (i.e., the capillary tube) is used to vary the gas to liquid ratio and thereby build different types of foam architectures inside a capillary. The capillary tube gives the food engineer control over the architecture of the foam.

[5] O Skurtys, P Bouchon, and JM Aguilera. 2008. Formation of bubbles and foams in gelatine solutions within a vertical glass tube. *Food Hydrocolloids* 22:706-714.

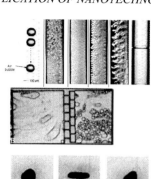

Architectures of foams made in a 250 μm coaxial capillary tube by varying the ratio gas/liquid flow rates (from Skurtys, Bouchon and Aguilera, 2007).

Oil droplets in an O/W emulsion after passage through a stack of layers of etched channels of a microfluidic device made from a silicon chip (from van der Zwan et al., 2006).

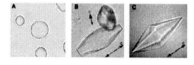

Evolution of a 2% potassium kappa-carrageenan particle subjected to capillary shearing flow during gelation (from Walther et al., 2004).

Different shapes of ice crystals made in: (A) Tris buffer; (B) Buffer and 400 mM of a polypeptide of an ice nucleating protein, and (C) Buffer and 50 mM of an anti-freeze protein (from Kobashigawa et al., 2005).

FIGURE 2-5 Four examples of reduced-size controlled structuring. For each example, the method or device that enables the controlled structuring is in **bold**. SOURCE: Reprinted from Food Hydrocolloids, Volume 22, Issue 4, O Skurtys, P Bouchon, and JM Aguilera, Formation of bubbles and foams in gelatine solutions within a vertical glass tube, pp. 706-714, Copyright (2008), with permission from Elsevier. E van der Zwan, K Schroën, K van Dijke, and R Boom, Visualization of droplet break-up in pre-mix membrane emulsification using microfluidic devices, pp. 223-229, Copyright (2006), with permission from Elsevier, Reprinted from Food Hydrocolloids, Volume 17, L Hamberg, M Wohlwend, P Walkenström, and A Hermansson, Shapes and shaping of biopolymer drops in a hyperbolic flow, pp. 641-652, Copyright (2008), with permission from Elsevier, Reprinted from FEBS Letters, Volume 579, Y Kobashigawa, Y Nishimiya, K Miura, S Ohgiya, A Miura, and S Tsuda, A part of ice nucleating protein exhibits the ice-binding ability, pp. 1493-1497, Copyright (2005), with permission from Elsevier; Reprinted from Colloids and Surfaces A: Physicochemical and Engineering Aspects.

2. Controlling a uniform size of oil droplets in an oil/water emulsion after passage through a stack of layers of etched channels of a *microfluidic device* made from a silicon chip.[6] Again, use of the micro-fluidic device gives the food engineer capacity to

---

[6] E van der Zwan, K Schroën, K van Dijke, and R Boom. 2006. Visualization of droplet break-up in pre-mix membrane emulsification using microfluidic devices. *Colloids and Surfaces A: Physicochemical and Engineering Aspects* 277:223-229.

manipulate food structure at a smaller size scale than has been possible in the past and at the size scale of the elements being formed.

3. Deforming particles of a 2 percent potassium kappa-carrageenan solution subjected to *capillary shearing flow* followed by *gelation.*[7] Capillary shearing enables the food engineer to shape soft materials into all sorts of odd shapes.

4. Different shapes of ice crystals made in (A) Tris buffer; (B) Buffer and 400 mM of a polypeptide of an *ice nucleating protein*; and (C) Buffer and 50 mM of an *anti-freeze protein.*[8] As Aguilera said, "Why not shape ice crystals? ... We could do that if we wanted...."

Food Microstructure and the Health/Nutrition Interface

Epidemiological data and other scientific evidence show an association between diet and the incidence of nutrition-related diseases. Aguilera identified three types of effects that contribute to this association:

1. Some nutrients and bioactive compounds have been shown *in vitro* to have specific beneficial health-related effects. Aguilera calls these isolated *in vitro* effects "specific effects."

2. Scientists have also found, however, that foods with the same basic composition can have different metabolic effects *in vivo* depending on the structure of the food. In other words, bioactive components perform differently in different structural matrices— Aguilera calls this the "matrix effect."

3. Moreover, because people tend to consume multiple foods at one time, added to this matrix effect are all of the various interaction effects that occur inside the digestive system. In other words, foods—not nutrients—are the key to understanding the nutrition-health interface in the body. Aguilera calls these "interaction effects."

---

[7] B Walther, L Hamberg, P Walkenström, and A-M Hermansson. 2004. Formation of shaped drops in a fast continuous flow process. *Journal of Colloid and Interface Science* 270:195-204.

[8] Y Kobashigawa, Y Nishimiya, K Miura, S Ohgiya, A Miura, and S. Tsuda. 2005. A part of ice nucleating protein exhibits the ice-binding ability. *FEBS Letters* 579:1493-1497.

There are plentiful opportunities to design new foods or modify existing ones to accommodate these three different types of effects with the goal of maintaining health and wellbeing. For example, the bioavailability of carotenoid compounds varies, depending on food matrix, with spinach having a very low bioavailability (with its "raw green leafy vegetable" matrix effect) and formulated natural or synthetic carotenoids have very high bioavailability (with their "when extracted and formulated as carotenoids in water-dispersible beadlets" matrix effect).

This variation raises the question, why? Why is the bioavailability of carotenoids from raw spinach, for example, so low? Why don't we get 100 percent of what we eat? There could be many reasons. For example, there may be a matrix effect (e.g., the nutrient may be entrapped in the matrix or complexed with macromolecules), or there may be an interaction effect when the food reaches the gut (e.g., the nutrient may get transformed into either a more or less active form once inside the gut, or it may interact with other food components once inside the gut).[9] Aguilera pointed to starch as a good example of how a single structural change induced by cooking can alter the health impact of a nutrient (see Figure 2-6). Starch is digested and converted into sugar, but the change in sugar concentration in the blood after eating a starch varies depending on whether and how long that starch has been cooked. Blood glucose levels increase more when the starch is cooked more.[10] So, cooking a starch can lead to very different glycemic responses. Moreover, the glycemic response varies depending on whether and how a single component interacts with other components, as is the case with food.[11] A different glycemic response would be expected for a simple carbohydrate, such as sugar, compared to a complex food such as bread, potatoes or spaghetti where starch, for example, interacts with other components in the mixture. Again, food structure affects nutrient impact.

---

[9] J Parada and JM Aguilera. 2007. Food microstructure affects the bioavailability of several nutrients. *Journal of Food Science* 72:R21-R32.

[10] J Parada and JM Aguilera. 2009. In vitro digestibility and glycemic response of potato starch is related to granule size and degree of gelatinization. *Journal of Food Science* 74:E34-E38.

[11] G Ricardi, G Clemente, and R Giacco. 2003. The importance of food structure in influencing postprandial response. *Nutrition Reviews* 61:S56-S60.

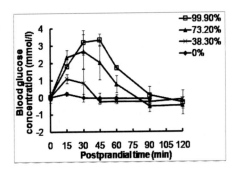

Glycemic response of potato starch samples having different degrees of gelatinization. Parada and Aguilera, 2008.

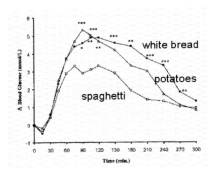

The importance of food structure in influencing postprandial response Ricardi, G., Clemente, G. & Giacco, R. Nutr. Rev. 61(5), S56-S60, 2003.

FIGURE 2-6 How food structure impacts glycemic response. The graph on the left illustrates how the blood glucose level is impacted by degree of gelatinization, with greater gelatinization (i.e., more cooking) causing a longer-lasting and high blood glucose level. The graph on the right illustrates how different foods cause different glycemic responses, depending on the structure of the food.

SOURCE: In vitro digestibility and glycemic response of potato starch is related to granule size and degree of gelatinization, J Parada and JM Aguilera. Copyright © 2009. Reproduced with permission of Blackwell Publishing Ltd.; Glycemic index of local foods and diets: the Mediterranean experience, G Ricardi, G Clemente, and R Giacco. Copyright © 2003. Reproduced with permission of Blackwell Publishing Ltd. [12]

Food Microstructure and the Gastronomy/Pleasure Interphase

Aguilera reminded the workshop audience that about one-third of the total food industry comprises food eaten outside the home; and that expenditures on "fine dining" are on the rise. He commented on how he has been working with many chefs over the last two years since, as he said, "chefs are the most creative and innovative people in the industry." Most of the 10 top chefs in the world today have their own molecular gastronomy laboratories. They love to experiment with new food

---

[12]Ibid.

structures and techniques. Also, as a reminder, some of the most famous food structures today are relatively young (e.g., mayonnaise is only about 200 years old). He encouraged food scientists to collaborate with some of these chefs, as there are many opportunities for innovation, including intervening at the micro- and nano-sized scales, and the dissemination of technologies.

Conclusion

Aguilera showed a graph diagramming the relative impacts and needs of nanoscience applications in foods and food processing and suggested that technologies/applications that create added values that are most needed and that will have the highest impact on consumers will be accepted first (see Figure 2-7). For example, added value with respect to making food processing more eco-friendly or making food safer will probably have the highest consumer impact and acceptability in the short term, would therefore be desirable to pursue. Health and well-being, designed functional foods, food protection, and tools to probe into the food microstructure are also high-need impact values. Applications of nanoscience to food processing by industry will also have a positive impact on consumers. Changes to food processing, on the other hand, are not as important with respect to the impact they would have on consumers. In this relative scale, foreign nanostructures added to foods, although needed in some cases, will have a lesser impact and can arouse negative perceptions on already well-fed consumers.

In conclusion, Aguilera emphasized three points:

1. If nanoscience and nanotechnology are defined as manipulating and assembling structures at the 1–100 nm level, then food processing has been doing it for centuries using many different types of molecules and processes although largely in an uncontrolled way.
2. Applications of novel micro- and nanotechnologies to food structuring are likely to bring large benefits to the food/health food industry. Examples of where this impact will be highest include the development of novel microprocesses, the creation of new textures and tastes, and the design of less calorie-dense foods with increased nutritional value and targeted nutrition for different lifestyles and conditions (e.g., obesity).

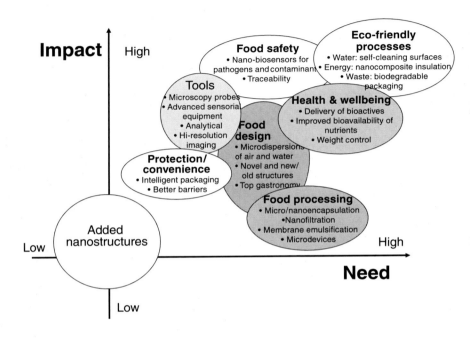

FIGURE 2-7 The impacts and needs of nanotechnology applications in foods and food processing. Shaded shapes are topics that Aguilera touched on during his talk. Image courtesy of José Miguel Aguilera.

3. But in order to do this, we need to increase our understanding of how existing food structures are formed and broken down, digested and absorbed. As we gain this better understanding, specific opportunities for nanosciences and nanotechnologies will become more apparent. If we do not gain this understanding, gaps in knowledge may lead to the delayed adoption of technologies and the inability to deal with risks and uncertainties.

MICRO AND NANOTECHNOLOGIES FOR
PROCESS CONTROL AND QUALITY
ASSESSMENT[13]

Presenter: Frans Kampers[14]

Kampers began by remarking that he would be discussing a topic that is not as controversial as some of the other topics being addressed during the course of this workshop: measurement and detection micro- and nanotechnologies. He emphasized that micro- and nanotechnologies will offer tremendous benefits not just within food products (i.e., by providing new types of food structures) but also *around* food products (e.g., through improved process control and quality assessment). In particular, he would be talking about micro- and nanotechnologies being developed for: (1) *sensing volatiles*, (2) *detecting microorganisms*, and (3) improving *packaging and product information*. Kampers described these nanotechnology applications as "low-hanging fruits." He said that focusing on these non-controversial, or less controversial, topics could provide a "stepping-stone for the general public to appreciate what nanotechnologies can offer to the food industry and where benefits for consumers can be derived from these technologies."

Sensing Volatiles: Building an Electronic Nose

Technologies that can sense volatiles rely on the use of receptor molecules that can adsorb small molecules that are released in certain monitored processes. Kampers explained how scientists at Wageningen UR are building "electronic noses" that can do just that and which are sensitive to certain volatiles. Basically, the noses are made of silicon crystal (i.e., a silicon chip) covered with an organic monolayer to which the receptors are bound; volatiles dock to the receptors, causing a charge shift that generates a signal in the silicon. At its simplest, the electronic

---

[13] This section is a paraphrased summary of Frans Kampers's presentation.

[14] Frans Kampers, PhD, co-coordinates research on nanotechnology in food, and he serves as Director, BioNT, Wageningen UR, The Netherlands. As Kampers explained during his presentation, Wageningen UR is both a university and contract research organization. It is one of the largest food and nutrition research organizations in the world. Its mission statement is "to explore the potential of nature and to improve the quality of life."

nose has a single receptor and single signal. Eventually, the Wageningen scientists would like to engineer an electronic nose with as many recaptors as the human nose contains. When we smell something, about 350 different receptors are activated, generating signals that our brain interprets—for example, whether a ham is "off" or not. Kampers's colleagues would like to build something that can do the same thing but electronically: a chip, or "electronic nose," that can derive information from and interpret the meaning of multiple signals.

One of the key challenges and one that nanotechnology can be used to address is making sure that the right receptors are on the right spots on the silicon chip. Using nanotechnology, one can "write addresses" on top of a chip by coating the chip with small single DNA strands, with each strand serving as an "address label." By linking complementary strands of DNA to particular receptor molecules, the receptors can find their own spots on the chip. Select the receptors that you would like the nose to contain, link complementary DNA molecules to them in a simple chemical procedure, wash those receptors over the DNA addresses, and ready is your very specific electronic nose. In a proof of principle experiment, Kampers and his colleagues used green fluorescent protein (GFP) to show that in fact they do bind to the appropriate place(s) on the chip.[15]

There are several potential applications of this nanotechnology-based electronic nose:

- Early detection of pests (e.g., early localization of pests in the greenhouse environment) which would help agricultural production.
- Monitoring and control (e.g., direct measuring of specific stages of a process such as a baking). Measuring volatiles would be more accurate than measuring temperature and time, which is how baking is monitored now and how product quality is controlled.
- Quality assurance (e.g., early warning in a refrigerated environment about whether a ham is no longer safe to eat).

---

[15] MA Jongsma and RH Litjens. 2006. Self-assembling protein arrays on DNA chips by auto-labeling fusion proteins with a single DNA address. *Proteomics* 6:2650-2655.

Microorganism Detection and Identification

Kampers described the potential applications of nanotechnology in the area of microorganism detection and identification as "very high impact," since for example as many as 2–4 million children in developing countries die every year of diarrhea-type diseases, any of which are contracted through food. Being able to detect what can and cannot be eaten is an important issue. In fact, the food industry has been doing a tremendous job at this. In industrialized countries, food has never been as safe as it is now. But obviously there is plentiful room for improvement. In the industrialized world, hospitalizations for and medical treatment of food illnesses exceeds several billion dollars per year. The success achieved to date is due in part to the functioning of food laboratories, where samples are incubated, pathogens detected and measured, and the status of raw materials readily determined. However, it often takes a day or two to get results from these laboratories. The food industry would like to speed up the process and be able to monitor processing much closer to the production line. So, for example, instead of waiting three days to know the status of a lot of precut lettuce, you would know it immediately. More specifically, the food industry is seeking small, handheld devices that can be operated by unskilled workers at the production site and that can derive information about the amount of pathogens or spoilage organisms on the food in a matter of minutes.

As one example, Kampers mentioned a nanotechnology-based lateral flow immunoassay device being developed by scientists at Wageningen. It is similar in principle, he said, to the lateral flow immunoassays used for pregnancy testing. It is a way of cheaply introducing that type of test, one that can detect specific DNA and produce results in a just a couple of minutes, into the armamentarium currently available to the food industry. Proof of principle studies have shown that the assay can accurately detect genetically modified soy and separate out genetically modified soy from wild type DNA soy.

In addition to GMO detection, the applications of this technology include:

- early detection of illness (e.g., in cows, which would be of enormous help to the dairy industry);
- traceability;

- food safety (e.g., detecting the number of spoilage organisms and predicting the shelf life of fresh fruit); and
- quality control.

Packaging and Information

Nanotechnology has already led to the availability of devices that detect a combination of temperature and time. For example, there are stickers that change color depending on the period and temperature at which a product has been stored, providing consumers with much more information about the quality of a product than "sell by" and other dates. Kampers showed a picture of such a sticker on meat packaging, with the color of the sticker indicating if the meat had been stored at a higher-than-acceptable temperature for over a certain period of time. Similar labels could be used to detect pathogens and micro-organisms. Kampers mentioned ToxicGuard™ and its use in the detection in food of *Listeria*, *Salmonella*, *E. coli*, and *Campylobacter*. Color-changing labels could also be used to detect ripeness. This is an interesting application, Kampers noted, since it is more about food quality than food safety. Different people prefer different types of apples, for instance people who are younger tend to prefer apples that are hard and a little sour, whereas people who are older tend to prefer soft, sweet apples; Kampers showed an image of a RipeSense label used with pears where a red dot means that the pear is crisp, a yellow dot that the pear is soft and sweet. So consumers could pick their flavors.

Radio frequency identification devices (RFID) could be used for similar purposes with the advantage that the information on the product can electronically be transferred from the product to devices in the logistical system, the shop, or even the refrigerator. Kampers said that RFID technology still requires a silicon chip as a substrate for the high frequency electronics and that it will probably be another decade or so before low-cost RFID for use with foods will be achievable. Scientists at Philips (an electronics company headquartered in Amsterdam, The Netherlands) are working on polymer-based RFIDs. When these technologies do become widely available in another 10–15 years, Kampers predicts that many food products will be labeled with RFID chips that can sense some kind of molecule and reveal directly to consumers what the status of the food product is and when (and when not) to consume the product.

USE OF NANOMATERIALS TO IMPROVE FOOD QUALITY AND FOOD SAFETY: NUTRIENT ENCAPSULATION AND FOOD PACKAGING[16]

Presenter: Jochen Weiss[17]

Weiss began by mentioning that he would be addressing one of the "more controversial" aspects of nanotechnology: using nanostructures as food ingredients (i.e., as opposed to using nanotechnology to engineer novel types of sensors and other non-food but food-related products). He said he would, however, briefly address the use of nanostructures in food packaging, noting that in fact one of the earliest applications of nano-structures in the food industry was the use of single-layer, clay-polymer composites in packaging, where single layers of clay are folded into a polymer system to create a new structure. These so-called exfoliated structures, or nanocomposites, prevent the passage of oxygen and water and have proven very stable to degradation. The U.S. Army, for example, is using this type of application to develop new packaging materials for ready-to-eat meals. Today, scientists like Julian McClements of the University of Massachusetts, Amherst, are taking this layering concept one step further and creating multi-layer food (not food packaging) droplets (i.e., microemulsions) and other food objects, where each layer is sequentially deposited onto the object, each layer giving that material a unique functionality (see Figure 2-8). So, for example, one could build a food material with antioxidant functionality in one layer, antimicrobial functionality in another layer, and the reduced passage of oxygen or water in yet another layer. Since the layers are nanometer thin, they would be invisible to the naked eye.

---

[16] This section is a paraphrased summary of Jochen Weiss's presentation.
[17] Jochen Weiss, PhD, is a Professor of Food Science and a Canada Research Chair in Food Protein Structure at the University of Guelph, Ontario.

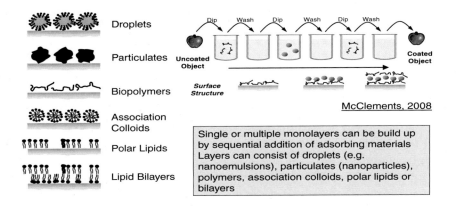

FIGURE 2-8 Julian McClements of the University of Massachusetts, Amherst, has been developing a method of adding multiple nanoscopic layers of functionalities to food objects. Starting materials can include droplets (microemulsions), particulates, biopolymers, association colloids, polar lipids or lipid bilayers.
SOURCES: IFT Status Summary: Nanotechnology-Applications in Food Processing and Product Development, J Weiss, P Takhistov, and DJ McClements. Copyright © 2006. *Journal of Food Science*. Reproduced with permission of Blackwell Publishing Ltd. Emulsion-based delivery systems for lipoliphic bioactive components, DJ McClements, J Weiss, and EA Decker. Copyright © 2007. *Journal of Food Sciences*. Reproduced with permission of Blackwell Publishing Ltd.[18]

Types of Nanomaterials and Nanostructures

There are several different types of functional nanostructures that can be used as building blocks to create novel structures and introduce new functionalities into foods, including: microemusions, liposomes, nanoemulsions, particles, fibers, and monolayers. Weiss described several of these structures, their actual and potential uses in the food industry, and research that he and his colleagues have been conducting with some of these various types of nano-sized materials.

---

[18] J Weiss, P Takhistov, and DJ McClements. 2006. IFT Status Summary: Nanotechnology–Applications in Food Processing and Product Development. *Journal of Food Science* 71(9):R107-R116. DJ McClements, J Weiss, and EA Decker. 2007. Emulsion-based delivery systems for lipoliphic bioactive components. *Journal of Food Science* 72(8):R109-R124. Reproduced with permission of Blackwell Publishing Ltd.

Microemulsions

Microemulsions are very, very small particles with diameters typically within the 5–50 nm range. Unlike emulsions, microemulsions are thermodynamically stable. They are transparent solutions, prepared by dispersing a milky solution and then adding some surfactants to the system; as such, they are actually three-component systems. They have a wide range of interesting applications. In non-food industries, they are used for enhanced oil recovery, in lubricants and coatings, and in cosmetics and agrochemicals. In the food industry AQUANOVA (a German supplier of liquid formulas), for example, makes a range of microemulsion products for solubilizing (i.e., increasing the water solubility of) important nutrients and vitamins. Microemulsions are also being explored for their potential to improve reaction efficiencies (e.g., interesterification, hydrogenation) and for fortification of foods.

Weiss and his colleagues are studying microemulsions for their potential to encapsulate and deliver antimicrobials. The researchers have shown that encapsulated concentrations of antimicrobials slow or completely stop *E. coli* growth in culture. When non-encapsulated anti-microbials are added, the antimicrobials partition into the aqueous phase only and there is not nearly as much bacterial inhibition. Encapsulated anti-microbials have also shown very high activity against bacterial biofilms, which are otherwise very resistant to disinfectants and difficult to remove from surfaces; unlike most disinfectants, which are typically inactivated in the top layer of a biofilm, because of their polymeric properties the microemulsions are able to penetrate down to the lower layers of the biofilm. Weiss said that when he and his colleagues started studying antimicrobial microemulsions, they built relatively simple systems, where they simply encapsulated an antimicrobial with a simple micelle. Since 2006, he and his team have been engineering more sophisticated antimicrobial carriers, by altering the surface properties of the micelle (i.e., by adding a charge and making an either anionic or cationic binary micelle) and then encapsulating the lipid antimicrobial with that altered, binary micelle. The charge gives the structure an electrostatic property that better targets microbial surfaces. Weiss explained how mixed microemulsions (e.g., mixed cationic/anionic micelles) are more stable than binary micelles in certain environments (e.g., cationic micelles are not very stable in refrigerated environments, but mixed cationic/nonionic micelles are).

The next step with microemulsions is to build even more complex structures, for example by combining charged binary microemulsions with charged food polymers, such as pectins, and creating stable microemulsion-polymer clusters with potentially improved functionalities) (see Figure 2-9). Weiss and his colleagues are experimenting with these more complex structures in an effort to make a palatable antimicrobial microemulsion (which would otherwise be too bitter to ingest).

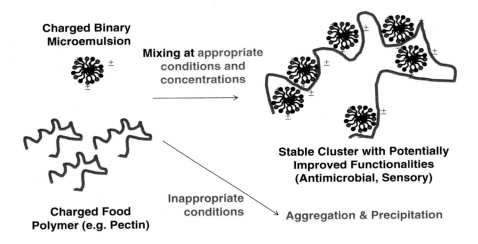

FIGURE 2-9 The next step for microemulsion nanotechnology is the creation of composite microemulsion-polymer clusters with novel functionalities, such as antimicrobial potency or palatability. Image courtesy of Jochen Weiss.

Liposomes

Liposomes are another type of nanostructure being used to add functionality to food. Liposomes are spherical bilayer membrane structures with aqueous cores, so unlike lipophilic-containing microemulsions, they can be used to contain and deliver hydrophilic, or water-soluble, ingredients. Moreover, their internal pH is adjustable, so they can contain ingredients that otherwise would not be stable under certain circumstances. As with microemulsions, there is a lot of engineering that can be done and different materials that can be used, leading to a range of differently shaped and sized final products. For example, depending on how the phospholipids base materials are put together, one could form either multiple vesicular structures or single onion-shaped vesicles. Also as with microemulsions, Weiss and his colleagues have been experimenting with liposomes as a way to encapsulate antibacterials, in this case nisin, and they have shown that encapsulated microemulsions are better than free nisin at inhibiting growth over a longer period of time, partly as a result of a more controlled and long-term sustained release.

Liposomes are, however, extremely fragile. A liposome is basically just a shell with water inside, and it leaks over time. In fact, this is why industry hasn't really been that interested in liposomes until now. Weiss and his colleagues have shown that it is possible to engineer leak-resistant liposome surfaces by surrounding the liposomes with polymeric layers and forming double-layered, or two-layer, liposomes. Two-layer liposomes are significantly more stable to long-term storage than single-layer liposomes, and they have greater controlled release possibilities (see Figure 2-10).

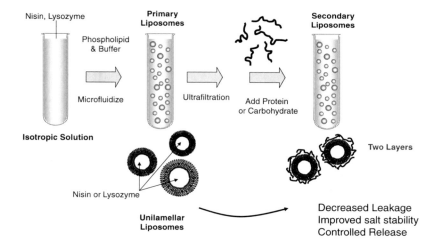

FIGURE 2-10 Next steps for nanoliposomes include forming double-layered liposomes ("secondary liposomes") that are more stable and leak-resistant than single-layer liposomes ("primary liposomes") and that have greater controlled release capabilities. Weiss and colleagues have been studying the capacity of liposomes to encapsulate and deliver antibacterials (i.e., nisin, lysozyme). Image courtesy of Jochen Weiss.

Biopolymeric Nanoparticles

Biopolymer nanoparticles are highly bioactive solid particles with diameters of 100 nm or less. They are already heavily used in the drug delivery industry, where they serve as the basis of modern anticancer drug delivery systems. Weiss and his colleagues have demonstrated that the particles can also serve as carriers of antimicrobial components, with nicin-containing biopolymeric nanoparticles exhibiting much more potent activity against *E. coli* O157:H7 than particles without nicin. The application of biopolymeric nanoparticles in the food industry is precluded however by the fact their manufacture requires the use of organic solvents. While alternative methods of assembly could be pursued, as of yet biopolymeric nanoparticles do not have any direct applications in food systems.

Solid Lipid Nanoparticles (SLNs)

An alternative to the biopolymer nanoparticle approach is the actual construction of solid particles using lipids as the base material. These so-called solid lipid nanoparticles, or SLNs, are basically crystallized emulsions composed of a high-melting point lipid and a bioactive lipophilic component. SLNs are typically about 50–500 nm in diameter and can be either sprayed or applied as powder. Smaller SLNs (i.e., 120–130 nm or less in diameter) have crystal structures that exhibit very different behaviors than those of larger SLNs because of surface-initiated crystallization. Because of these behaviors, smaller SLNs serve as highly effective carrier systems for susceptible bioactive ingredients. Weiss and his colleagues have demonstrated this fact by showing that SLN-encapsulated β-carotene lasts much longer than nonencapsulated β-carotene when stored at 20°C. Interfacial engineering is the key to success. When the interfaces of the SLNs are not engineered properly, the emulsions degrade very rapidly and the β-carotene is lost very quickly over storage time. If, however, the engineering of the SLN interface is done properly (i.e., via surface-initiated crystallization using saturated lecithin as the surfactant), the resultant crystal structure readily entraps the β-carotene and with very little degradation over the time.

The next step forward, Weiss said, is the creation of more complex structures. He pointed to the work of David Weitz, Harvard University, who has shown how SLNs can be used to form shells around emulsion droplets, creating what are known as colloidosomes. As with simpler SLNs, colloidosomes can be loaded with bioactive compounds, which are released upon the application of mechanical or thermal stress.

Nanofibers

Finally, Weiss described some of the work he and his colleagues have been doing with nanofibers. He explained how the fibers are produced through a process known as electrospinning, whereby an electric voltage is applied to a polymer solution, resulting in deposits of either microparticles or very ultra fine fibers. The fibers range in size from 30–500 nm in diameter. The advantage to this technique is that a variety of morphologies of particles can be created, with different morphologies having different properties and textural attributes. As they have with other types of nanomaterials, Weiss and his colleagues have demonstrated that nanofiber technology can be used to create potent antimicrobial systems that maintain their antimicrobial capacity for long periods of time. In collaboration with researchers at the University of Tennessee, Weiss and colleagues have also demonstrated how nanofibers serve as ideal materials for catalysis because of their extremely high surface-to-mass ratio and high reaction kinetics. By modulating the surface, some very unusual reactions can be run that would not be possible with larger structures.

Future steps include combining nanofibers with other nano-scale systems, namely microemulsions, and building more complex structures with greater functionalities (see Figure 2-11). Weiss and his colleagues have demonstrated that the technique of co-spinning antimicrobial microemulsions inside the nanofibers can yield another type of highly active antimicrobial nanofiber system.

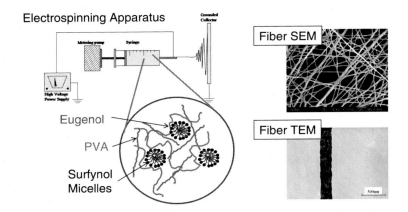

FIGURE 2-11 One of the next steps with nanofiber technology in food is to combine the nanofibers with others type of nanomaterials, in this case microemulsions, to form novel structures with new functionalities. Image courtesy of Jochen Weiss.

The Future of Nanoscience: Playing Lego with Molecules

In conclusion, Weiss said that it is difficult to predict the future direction of nanoscience, since many of these structures are being built faster than their new properties (and potential functionalities) can be determined. However, what we have learned so far has allowed us to begin experimenting with architectural design and creating new microscopic structures with this wide range of simple building blocks. The building blocks can be combined in various ways (e.g., microemulsions inside of nanofibers), giving us enormous control over how these systems are assembled.

In contrast to how food structures have traditionally been constructed (i.e., from recipes), nanoscience enables a bottom-up design approach using molecules as the starting material: We then assemble these molecules and engineer their surfaces in ways that lead to new functionalities. We do not fully understand, however, how most of these structures are going to function within the food matrix where they will be applied. Many unanswered questions remain about their lifetime, mobility, and location inside actual food systems. Understanding this complex interaction between the nanostructures and the food products that contain them is critical to discussing safety.

OPEN DISCUSSION[19]

Following Weiss's presentation, there was a 20-minute open question and answer period. While most of the questions revolved around the actual science and technology of nanostructured food, workshop participants also asked about regulatory uncertainty around food nanotechnology. More specifically, questioners asked about when the potential applications of food nanotechnology will be realized and commercially available; whether and how regulatory uncertainty around food nanotechnology is impacting corporate investment and intention to bring these products to market; whether and how the definition and history of nanotechnology (-ies) play into some of the unanswered questions around regulation; whether and how nanotechnology is being used to address the palatability issues typically associated with nutrient delivery; and whether there are limitations to food nanotechnology such that smaller might not always be better.

When Will These Opportunities Be Realized?

Doyle opened the discussion with a question about the short-term opportunities among all of the various and very exciting applications that were described throughout the morning. Weiss, Kampers, and Aguilera all offered responses. Weiss stated that the applications revolving around the delivery of functional ingredients will be immediate and that, in fact, some of the simpler systems have been available for quite a while. He cited AQUANOVA's encapsulated bioactive products as one example. However, some composite structures currently being researched and developed, such as those that he described during his presentation, are longer-term prospects.

Kampers concurred that some encapsulated food nanotech products are already on the market. However, the food industry does not refer to these products as "nanotechnology," even though scientists classify them

---

[19] This section is a paraphrased summary of the open discussion that followed Weiss talk.

as nanostructure materials. Also, many of the measurement, sensor, and diagnostic applications currently in development, such as those that he described during his presentation, are very close to being market ready.

Aguilera commented that those applications that can satisfy consumer needs unmet by traditional or conventional items would reach the market first. Weiss agreed with Aguilera, stating additionally that consumer benefit, not the potential to decrease company costs, company cost-cutting, "should be the main driver" of nanotechnology. This last comment prompted an unidentified audience member to state that a good business strategy should be able to balance consumer demand with company cost-cutting efforts.

Another unidentified audience member then asked Kampers about the time frame of commercialization for a specific application that Kampers described: the early detection of volatiles. Specifically, when will this technology be available for refrigerators and packaging? Kampers said that technologies are already available for the detection of volatiles in air and that nanotechnology is simply increasing the specificity and sensitivity of this type of detection. He predicts that these improvements will probably be achieved within the next five years.

Corporate Intent and Regulatory Uncertainty

An unidentified workshop attendee remarked that there has been "pull back" in industry because of high early expectations for nanotechnology that remain unmet. The questioner then asked, what is the current level of corporate investment and intention to bring these various applications to market, and how does regulatory uncertainty affect that? Weiss responded first by saying that the investment and intention still exist but that much of what happens in the food industry happens "behind closed doors." There are a lot of intellectual property rights riding on many of these developments. Also, as with any emerging technology, these types of applications take many years of development before products are ready to enter the market. Moreover, also like any new technology, nanotechnology solves existing problems in many cases, but it also creates new challenges and requires optimizing.

Kampers agreed with Weiss and added that regulation is definitely an issue since industry views regulation as something that limits the possibilities. On the other hand, regulation is critical to building trust with consumers and ensuring that the public accepts the technology. With good regulation in place, consumers recognize the presence of an objective body that is maintaining some sort of control over applications of the new technology. Without good regulation, consumers must rely on the industry itself. He said that this lack of regulation and absence of an objective body responsible for maintaining control "might be the key element that is missing in the current situation."

Definition and History of Nanotechnology: More Questions About Regulatory Uncertainty

Food Forum member Ned Groth commented on Aguilera's discussion of the definition of nanotechnology. He said that food has been engineered for a long time in ways "involving molecules" and that the main difference between what has been done in the past and what is now being done with nanotechnology seems to be that the latter involves doing things on a "smaller scale." Nanotechnology allows us to combine the natural components of foods in more useful ways than has been done in the past, but it is still part of a continuum of the engineering of components. In contrast, genetically modified foods created through recombinant DNA technology represented a sharp line between the "old, traditional science" and modern biotechnology. While societies have been cross-breeding and genetically improving animals and plants for a long time, genetically modified organism (GMO) technology enabled the introduction of genetic combinations, like salmon and tomato DNA, that do not naturally exist. Groth asked, "Can you draw such a line [with nanotechnology in food]? Is there a way to separate what would be a novel introduction of technology at a nano-level?" In particular, is there a way to delineate at what point the use of nanotechnology "might raise some concerns and therefore be subject to more intense regulatory oversight" compared to the current standard for products derived from traditional food science?

Kampers replied that the definition of nanotechnology (in food) is "very, very difficult," and yet a definition is necessary for regulation. Regulation, in turn, is necessary to control risks. Kampers identified persistent, non-dissolvable, non-biodegradable nanoparticles as the predominant source of food nanotechnology risks. He emphasized that most nanotechnology does not involve nanoparticles and that most nanoparticles are naturally existing, not synthetic, materials.

Aguilera reiterated some of the comments he had made during his presentation. He mentioned that he did not recall ever having read anything explaining to consumers that the food industry has been operating within the nano-range for a long time and that it would be interesting for consumers to realize this. He referred to the examples he described during his presentation (e.g., dairy technology revolves around the use of milk proteins, fat globules and casein micelles, all of which can be measured in nanometers). However, until recently, the food industry hasn't actually targeted objects at the nano-scale when working with food structure since it was widely believed that most functionalities and properties of food were determined by objects within the 1–100 μm range (i.e., the micrometer, not nanometer range). Now, food scientists are realizing that the assembly of these smaller objects is important and that there is still a lot of work to be done with respect to understanding how even naturally existing nano-sized objects in conventional foods give foods their properties.

Later during the discussion, there was another, related question about what the questioner said was a lack of clear distinction between nano and micro, especially in food, and whether and how the "infiltration" of "nano" can be detected. The questioner commented that manipulation at the micro scale is generally accepted (and implied that manipulation at the nano scale is not generally accepted). Kampers responded by saying that he, for one, is "not very particular" about the distinction since the goal is to create new functionality; whether that new functionality is created by manipulating below 100 nm (at the nano level) or above 100 nm (at the micro level) is not the issue.

Palatability

The discussion shifted back toward issues about the technology itself. Van Hubbard from the NIH commented that one of the reasons he and his group[20] were interested in this workshop was to gain a better understanding of how nanotechnology can be used to improve health. He mentioned that one of the issues addressed during the morning session, nutrient delivery, touched on this theme. One of the issues with nutrient delivery, in turn, is palatability. He asked the panel to comment on the

---

[20] Hubbard is the Director of the NIH Division of Nutrition Research Coordination, which is housed within the National Institute of Diabetes and Digestive and Kidney Diseases, or NIDDK.

use of nanotechnology to address the issue of palatability. Specifically, how can nanotechnology be used to introduce critical nutrients into the food supply in such a way that those ingredients are bioavailable and the foods still palatable?

Weiss agreed that palatability is a major issue with nutrients. When nutrients are added to foods, the flavor or textural attributes of the food are often compromised. Weiss referred to the antimicrobial examples he gave during his presentation (i.e., adding antimicrobial components to various types of nanomaterials), commenting that adding antimicrobials to foods creates the same palatability problem. "While it's a wonderful compound," he said, "you can't apply them in a product without the consumer rejecting them." He said that efforts to engineer products with functionalities that change the way the products interact with the taste receptors on the tongue, for example, would have an impact on palatability.

Kampers agreed with Weiss, stating that one of the new functionalities that nanotechnology can deliver is the capacity to control where in the human body an encapsulate will fall apart and release its nutrient or other contents. In cases where the nutrient contents of the encapsulate do not taste good, the encapsulate could be engineered not to break apart until it reached the small intestine, for example, where it would have the greatest effect anyway. As a second example, Kampers mentioned that Nestlé has developed an encapsulated product filled with both vitamin A and iron and engineered so that both ingredients don't become available until they reach the wall of the gastrointestinal (GI) tract, where their combined availability is necessary for absorption. He referred to studies in Morocco that have shown how the addition of nanoencapsulated iron to salt can reduce iron deficiency in children.

Aguilera added that the issue of palatability is a difficult one, since it involves human biology of the brain as well as mouth, but that there have been reports linking the structure and shape of small particles to tongue sensation. He reiterated that correlating people's responses to food manipulations at the nanoscale is a new area of study which scientists have been investigating for only the last 8–10 years.

Is Small Always Better?

Food Forum member Eric Decker of the University of Massachusetts, Amherst, commented on the very exciting applications discussed throughout the morning. "I didn't hear the other side of it. Are there some limitations?" he asked. "Is smaller always going to be better?" In particular, by manipulating at this very small scale, one dramatically increases bioavailability—is that a risk? Is there a risk to stability? Where is nanotechnology *not* going to work?

Kampers agreed that, yes, there are risks, not just with the nanoparticles themselves but with other components of the system for which nanotechnology serves simply as "the deliverer." Consider bioavailability. What if a consumer eats two or three different products, each with very high bioavailability of a given nutrient? What are the consequences of that? Those consequences would not directly be related to the nanotechnology, but nanotechnology makes them possible and therefore they are risks we must consider.

Weiss agreed that Decker raised a very important point. He said, "I do not agree with the statement 'small is always better'; definitely not." He said that sometimes nanotechnology will improve food products, but other times it will not, and "we need to critically evaluate in which cases we gain clear benefits and derive clear new functionalities that are good. If we don't see those benefits, we are much better off staying with the systems we have, which are microstructured systems where we have a lot of experience." He urged everybody involved with food structure development to critically examine their structures and identify where and how those structures would be useful, recognizing that not all nanostructures will be "good."

Related to the issue of risk, Doyle asked whether the antimicrobial applications that Weiss and his colleagues were studying would impact the gut microflora once inside the human body. "What's that going to do to the gut flora when you consume a long-lasting antimicrobial component?" Doyle asked. Weiss responded, "There is absolutely the possibility that you can impact the microflora." Fortunately, he said, target specificity can be built into these systems, and that will likely be an area of active future research.

3

Safety and Efficacy of Nanomaterials in Food Products

This chapter summarizes the presentations and discussion that took place during the second session of the workshop. The first presenter, Martin Philbert of the University of Michigan, argued that scientists do not fully understand all of the safety issues associated with nanotechnology. He emphasized that in addition to thinking about the nanosized materials themselves, it is important to consider all of the "things that come along with the nanotechnology." As examples, he pointed to the biocompatible surfactants often added to nanoparticles as a way to prevent clumping and the metals that are sometimes used during the synthesis of carbon nanotubes: both of these added substances raise potential toxicity issues. It is also important to consider how nanomaterials behave not just in the context of the food matrix (which Aguilera had previously addressed) but also in the context of the biological size scale (i.e., inside the human body). After commenting on some of what is already known about the toxicity of nanomaterials, Philbert briefly described some recent toxicity studies and then identified several key safety issues that remain unresolved.

The second presenter, Laura Tarantino of the U.S. Food and Drug Administration (FDA), provided an overview of the range of FDA authorities over food products and argued that nanotechnology can be viewed as a special case of what the FDA has been doing all along with food. Essentially, the burden of proof is on manufacturers to show that any changes they have made do not affect safety. The challenge is determining what types of testing and data are necessary for determining this. FDA has yet to issue formal guidance for nanotechnology in food, and Tarantino encouraged sponsors who are considering developing nanomaterials-based products to engage in early and frequent consultation with the agency. Not only would early consultation benefit manufacturers, by providing them with an indication of what types of testing and data would be required for approval, it would also provide the FDA with information that could be helpful as it develops the necessary guidance.

The third and final speaker of this session, Fred Degnan of King & Spaulding, broached some of the same issues that Tarantino did, but as Degnan put it, "from a practicing lawyer's perspective." He agreed with Tarantino that the FDA's statutory authorities provide the agency with the necessary tools for evaluating and regulating the safety of nanomaterials with novel properties and that the FDA's existing procedures and systems are adequate to evaluate and regulate nanotechnology in food. In fact, the Food Additive Amendment (FAA) of 1958, which was enacted in response to a post-WWII public health scenario created by the sudden availability of thousands of new synthetic chemicals, was designed to address the very same types of safety issues presented by the use in food of nanomaterials with novel properties. However, he argued that the basis of good regulation is in written guidance, not just "chatting" (to borrow Tarantino's expression). Any type of written guidance, even if preliminary, would be of enormous benefit, not just for improving industry understanding but also for ensuring public confidence that FDA is engaged and focused on nanotechnology issues. This is particularly true of nanomaterials introduced into food products that have previously been exempt from premarket approval because they are Generally Recognized as Safe (GRAS).

Again, there was an open discussion period at the end of the session. Most of the questions pertained to issues around toxicology and whether there are any established criteria for how to proceed; how to encourage early industry consultations with the FDA; whether there is an approximate timeline for when the FDA will be providing written guidance pertaining to nanomaterials with novel properties in food products; and under what, if any, circumstances a food designed to deliver nutrients can and should be considered a drug for the purposes of regulation.

A BIOLOGICAL PERSPECTIVE ON
NANOSTRUCTURES IN FOODS[1]

Presenter: Martin A. Philbert[2]

Philbert began by remarking: "We are in the realm right now of almost infinite possibilities and very few probabilities." While it is easy to see in the laboratory or "boutique" commercial setting a variety of interesting, novel nano-structures with all sorts of desirable properties, turning nanotechnology into a "useful iteration that can be safely deployed into a human body is a very different proposition." There are a wide range of safety issues that need to be considered. Importantly, in addition to thinking about the toxicity of the nanomaterial itself, he said, "We need to pay very close attention to those things that we add in order to deploy the nanotechnology appropriately. And in fact, the nanotechnology itself may be a bit of a misdirect in that really what we're looking at is toxicity of things that come along with the nanotechnology."

For example, consider that one of the fundamental properties of nanoparticles is the inverse relationship between particle size and the number of molecules expressed on the surface. As the diameter of a nanoparticle decreases the surface area increases; when particle diameter reaches the nanoscale level (< 100 nm) the ratio of surface molecules expressed increases exponentially. Below 100 nm, forces that are virtually negligible in the bulk scale begin to predominate (e.g., hydrogen bonding, van der Walls forces, and other interactions that tend to drive particles together). Philbert described the results of a study published in *Science* (Nel et al., 2006) showing more generally how dose metrics become more complex as size decreases (i.e., this is true not just of nanoparticles but all types of nanomaterials).[3] For example, when carbon nanotubes are taken out of pristine deionized water and placed in solution, they tend to agglomerate very quickly because of the forces that predominate at these smaller sizes. Biocompatible surfactants can be added as a way to prevent agglomeration, but they present their own set of challenges.

---

[1] This section is a paraphrased summary of Martin Philbert's presentation.
[2] Martin A. Philbert, PhD, is Professor of Environmental Sciences and Associate Dean for Research at University of Michigan's School of Public Health.
[3] A Nel, T Xia, L Mädler, and N Li. 2006. Toxic potential of materials at the nanolevel. *Science* 311:622-627.

The addition of biocompatible surfactants is an example of why close attention needs to be directed not just to the toxicity of the nanomaterial itself (e.g., the carbon nanotube) but also to "those things that we add in order to deploy the nanotechnology appropriately." Another example, Philbert said, is the use of metals such as indium, vanadium, and sometimes technetium during the synthesis of carbon nanotubes and the consequent, unintended delivery of a very reactive metal during the delivery of the therapeutic to a biological setting.

Also in addition to considering the toxicity of all of the various added substances required to deploy a nanotechnology application appropriately, one must consider what happens to the nanomaterial in the biological context. Philbert pointed to some very interesting studies coming out of Dublin[4] that show how durable carbonaceous materials, when introduced into a high protein environment such as the inside of a cell, can cause abnormal protein fibrillation. (Fibrillation is the formation of fibrils; amyloid protein fibrillation is a type of aggregation phenomena that has been linked to many human diseases.) This may be of some consequence in individuals who are either genetically predisposed to or already have the equivalent of familial amyloidosis (a protein-misfolding disease); the nanomaterial may act as a seed around which the amyloid proteins aggregate.

Nanomaterials Are Here: Factual and Fanciful

From C_{60} buckminsterfullerenes (spherical structures composed of carbon atoms) to dendrimers (structure with repeatedly branching molecules), nanomaterials are here, and they are being used in all sorts of "sublime" but also controversial ways. For example, novel metals and metal oxides are being encapsulated for the enhancement of color and the imparting of beautiful shimmering effects on the surfaces of cars, aircrafts, etc. As another example, nanosized titanium dioxides and zinc oxides are being incorporated into sunscreens, allowing people to stay in the sun 60 times longer than they can with sunscreens with chemical additives, preventing burns and decreasing the likelihood of developing basal cell carcinoma down the line. Philbert noted that the use of these sunscreens raises questions about potential adverse health effects associ-

---

[4] E.g., S Linse, C Cabaleiro-Lago, W-F Xue, I Lynch, S Lindman, E Thulin, SE Radford, and KA Dawson. 2007. Nucleation of protein fibrillation by nanoparticles. *Proceedings of the National Academy of Sciences* 104:8691-8696.

ated with entry of the nanomaterials into the human body. For the home, you can now buy nano-based windows and wood floors. And finally, in health care, nanotechnology is being used to develop targeted delivery of therapeutics; Philbert pointed to the work of Donald Tomalia[5] as one example of an application; targeting therapeutics to cancer cells.

One needs to be very careful, Philbert said, about the claims being made about nanotechnology, as these claims very quickly go "from the sublime to the ridiculous." As just one example, there are "plans afoot" to add a nano-structured robot to the back of a spermatozoon, raising questions about the ethical implication of "subverting normal biological processes and achieving something that nature never intended to occur."

Moreover, not all that claims to be nanotechnology is truly "nano." There are now more than 800 self-identified nanotechnology products on the market. "Self-identified" is the key word. In fact, it is not really clear how many products on the market actually contain nanomaterials, Philbert said. They range from nanosilver-containing socks that people can wear for seven days without any appreciable odor to stain-resistant pants and ties. But then there are things like the iPod nano, a great example of a "nano" product that has nothing to do with "nano" except perhaps for the micro-circuitry (which Philbert said is irrelevant from a consumer perspective since consumers are never exposed to it).

Of those products that are coming on the market, many contain Nano-Ag^0 ("Nano-Silver") and other nanomaterials designed to come into contact with food. The life cycle of these composite materials is unknown, for example whether repeated dishwashing will "re-liberate" the nanomaterial despite the fact that there are physical forces that pull against that (i.e., once the material is embedded in a resin, it requires a great deal of energy to liberate the nanoparticle as a nanomaterial).

Evaluating the Safety of Nanomaterials

Philbert differentiated between risk and the perception of risk. He reminded the audience that risk is a product of hazard times exposure, which means that very few people are likely to be exposed to many of these products (especially because these materials are expensive). He showed an image of a person titrating an aerosolized nanomaterial and commented that while the worker is potentially exposed most consumers

---

[5] Tomalia is the Scientific Director of the National Dendrimer and Nanotechnology Center, Central Michigan University, Mt. Pleasant, MI.

of the product containing this particular nanomaterial aren't exposed to the actual nanomaterial. Rather, the risk for them is the greater force of impact resulting from a collision with a five-ton truck with nanoengineered high-tensile strength bumpers. "Where here is the greater risk?" Philbert asked. The potential health risks extend beyond exposure to the nanomaterial itself and include exposure to the final engineered products as well. He said, "I urge all of us to think more broadly about the implication of the inclusion into materials, not just the hazard associated with limited exposure to material."

Current Knowledge of Nanoscale Material Toxicity

Knowledge about physical properties of other materials can be used to predict how nanoparticles will behave and whether they will be toxic in the human body. For example, some formulations of long and thin nanotubes would probably behave like asbestos, depending on the biological and physical context, since both materials have high aspect (length:width) ratios. Other properties with known toxicities include biopersistence, the presence of reactive surfaces or points (i.e., areas capable of producing reactive oxygen species), certain compositions, and solubility. For example, manganese in welding fume produces an aerosol of particles, most of which are under 100 nm in diameter, and it is well known that many welders develop manganism as a result of this exposure. (Manganism is similar to Parkinson disease, with various part's of the brain that control motor movement degenerating.) As another example, the cadmium, selenium, and arsenic in quantum dots are soluble at physiological pH; so while a quantum dot may have great functionality, it also serves as a delivery device for super-physiological concentrations of cadmium. While coating some of these potentially toxic materials with biocompatible substances (with dextran, titanium oxide, zinc oxide, or polyethylene glycol) can significantly reduce toxicity, it does not obviate all of the toxicity.

Size Is Not Everything

Philbert emphasized, "Size is not everything." There is a tendency to think that all brand new nanomaterials are "bad," but there are other factors besides size to consider before passing judgment. He described unpublished data showing that injecting even a ridiculously high dose of nanomaterial into the tail vein of a rat over the course of an hour, say 500 mg per kg, which he likened to injecting "cottage cheese," has no patho-logical consequences (if the material can be injected without inducing any hydrodynamic changes). However, if the same nanomaterial carrier is used to deliver iron into a different biological context, namely the re-nal cortex and liver, the result is cortical renal necrosis and petechial hemorrhage (a subcutaneous hemorrhage occurring in minute spots) in the liver. So again, size is not the only factor to consider when evaluating safety.

Moreover, there is considerable variation in size among nanoparti-cles even in a single system. An carbon nanotube (CN) aerosolized, for example, contains particles ranging in size from smaller than 0.01 μm to greater than 1 μm in diameter. When the aerosol is agitated, the propor-tion of particles smaller than 100 nm increases drastically.

Toxicity Studies

Philbert described the results of a toxicity study that involved expos-ing mice to a variety of concentrations of aerosolized CNs, demonstrat-ing that CNs can cause inflammatory disease and destruction in the lungs with widespread formation of granulomas.[6] Based on data from studies like this, it is well known now that a variety of nanomaterials interact with the immune system to produce effects ranging from mild stimula-tion of the immune system to severe granulomatous change in, for in-stance, the lung.

It is important, however, to make sure that these experiments are done properly and that the properties of the nanomaterial do not, as Philbert said, "defeat the experimental design." Philbert showed a light micrograph image of lung tissue from a rat exposed to 5 mg/kg of single-walled carbon nanotube (SWCNT). After only a few hours of exposure, the rats in this experiment started dying but not because of pulmonary toxicity; rather, they suffocated because their airways had been mechanically blocked by the SWCNT instillate. So in that case, the death and destruction had "nothing to do with nano." In fact, if you disperse the SWCNT instillate appropriately, rather than suffocation, you see a progressive granulomatous disease.

When "assigning blame in the context of toxicology," Philbert said, you also have to be very careful about which particle, or rather which

---

[6] The image and graph were Figure 1 in C-W Lam, JT James, R McCluskey, and RL Hunter. 2004. Pulmonary toxicity of single-wall carbon nanotubes in mice 7 and 90 days after intratracheal instillation. *Toxicological Sciences* 77:126-134.

particle shape, is the culprit. Even a single nanotube can have multiple morphologies.[7] Is the damage being caused by the smaller nanotubes, the larger ones, or multimers of differently shaped nanotubes? Most commercial preparations are mixtures of morphologies, with the goal of increasing tensile strength for less cost, so very rarely are pure samples being prepared in bulk.

Despite the lack of clarity around what exactly is causing the damage, it appears that some organs, namely the liver, spleen, and lymph nodes, tend to accumulate nanomaterial much more quickly than other organs do. One could inadvertently concentrate a nanomaterial in these organs while targeting other tissues in the body. The liver, for instance, contains Kupffer cells (a specialized type of macrophage located in the liver and forms part of the reticuloendothelial system), which line the sinusoidal wall and are responsible for removing toxins from the blood entering the liver from the gut mesentery. The Kupffer cells normally pick up small viruses and infectious particles, which are in the nano range (i.e., less than 100 nm), and so they presumably pick up other nano-sized substances as well. Philbert mentioned a 2006 study published in the *Proceedings of the National Academy of Science (PNAS)* showing that no immediate adverse health effects were found after injecting individualized CNs directly into the bloodstream of rabbits.[8] The nanotubes circulated in the blood for more than an hour before being removed by the liver. Philbert argued that having "unmodified CNs cleared by the liver" is not necessarily a good thing; while "it is good pharmacokinetically and maybe even toxicokinetically," having these long-lived materials in the liver could be harmful.

Nanomaterials and the Biological Size Scale

Another important feature of nanomaterials with respect to safety is that they fall within the biological size scale. Indeed, this is why they have so many potential applications—nanomaterials can interact with biological components with very high affinity. For example, you can

---

[7] MS Arnold, AA Green, JF Hulvat, SI Stupp, and MC Hersam. 2006. Sorting carbon nanotubes by electronic structure using density differentiation. *Nature Nanotechnology* 1:60-65.

[8] P Cherukuri, CJ Gannon, TK Leeuw, HK Schmidt, RE Smalley, SA Curley, and RB Weisman. 2006. Mammalian pharmacokinetics of carbon nanotubes using intrinsic near-infrared fluorescence. *Proceedings of the National Academy of Sciences* 103:18882-18886.

now purchase kits for CN-based methods for isolating nucleic acids: the method works because a nucleic acid phospholipid wraps around a carbon nanotube so readily.[9] But that same affinity can be damaging. For example, work from Philbert's lab suggests that an array of proteins, including apolipoprotein A, can readily stick to the surfaces of the coated nanoparticles (e.g., nanoparticles coated with wheat germ agglutinin) that are being developed as a novel mode of drug delivery. Apolipoprotein A is involved with the transport of lipids into the brain and also with some parts of the oxygenation cascade—its attraction to these coated nanoparticles, Philbert said, "may or may not lead to inflammatory damage."

Philbert briefly addressed the issue of whether nanomaterials can penetrate the skin. He referred to work on quantum dots being done by Sally Tinkle of the National Institute of Environmental Health Sciences (NIEHS) and Paul Howard and others at the FDA. Tinkle has shown that quantum dots can penetrate flexed and stretched skin; Howard has shown the same with abraded skin. Also, nanoparticles can clearly penetrate cut skin, which Philbert said has implications for kids at the beach who are wearing nanoparticle-based sunscreen—if they have scuffed knees, for example, those nanoparticles are going to enter their bodies. Translocation (of just nanoparticles or both quantum dots and nanoparticles?) across the skin is always to the proximal lymph node, but it is unclear whether there is any lymphadenopathy as a result. There is no evidence yet of lymphadenoapathy, despite a long history of introducing fine and ultra-fine materials into the skin (e.g., tattooing).

Unpublished research in Philbert's lab shows that, as the dose of introduced nanomaterial increases, a greater fraction of that dose resides in "interstitial state" tissue. That is, there are mechanisms that he and his colleagues do not quite yet understand that suggest that introduced nanomaterials are picked up by the liver and other major immune system organs but then diffuse through the tissue(s) such that their exact cellular location cannot be pinpointed.

One of these (other) major immune system organs is the gut, specifically the Peyer patches (and M cells, which is where the Peyer patches attach to the gut) and dendritic cells. The M and dendritic cells take part in the constant "sampling" of the microflora of the gut and are involved

---

[9] Y Wu, JS Hudson, Q Lu, JM Moore, AS Mount, AM Rao, E Alexov, and PC Ke. 2006. Coating single-walled carbon nanotubes with phospholipids. *Journal of Physical Chemistry B* 110:2475-2478.

with mechanisms that promote a healthy flora.[10] Philbert stated that since "not all guts are 'normal,' it would be foolish for us to assume that all interactions of nanomaterials in food are going to be utterly predictable." Not only is there wide variation in gut microflora, but also there is wide variation in the "tone" of the epithelium of the gut, with the morphology of the gut lining changing with microfloral composition.

In conclusion, Philbert summarized the following:

- Dosimetry for nanomaterials is not clear. Do we measure mass concentration, surface area, chemical identity, chemical dose, or some complex algorithm that incorporates all of these factors?

- We are in "desperate need" of accurate quantitative methods for measuring nanomaterials in complex media such as food. There is an assumption that when we put a nanomaterial in food, it is going to remain a nanomaterial, but we have yet to confirm that this is true.

- The long-term stability of nano-enabled products is unknown. We "sort of know intuitively" that our food naturally breaks down into nanomaterials before being absorbed (since the "machines of life" operate at the nanoscale), but we do not know what happens to these nanomaterials as they pass through various media, including after they are eliminated from the body. In fact, environmentally deposited nanomaterials may be reintroduced into the food chain at a later point; life cycle analysis is important.

- Quantitative absorption, distribution, metabolism, and excretion (ADME) models are unavailable for most nanomaterials. Consider the C_{60} buckyball. If you were to add a hydroxyl group to it, there are 59! [59 factorial = $1 \times 2 \times 3 \times \ldots \times 59$] possible positions for the next hydroxyl group, 58! for the next, and so on. We will never have the resources or time to do an exhaustive toxicology on all of these new nanomaterials. Philbert said, "We need to put our collective thinking caps on and come up with a rational approach that is resource-appropriate for the identification of hazards and

---

[10] See J-P Kraehenbuhl and M Corbett. 2004. Keeping the gut microflora at bay. *Science* 303:1624-1625.

the establishment of risk and, ultimately, the management of risk."

- We need to know the impact of nanomaterials on non-pulmonary systems and determine whether or not the immune system effects that have been done in non-gastrointestinal (GI) systems translate to these other systems.

- We need to better understand both the acute and chronic effects of nanomaterials on the immune system. We are gathering data on the former, but virtually nothing is known about the latter. We need to develop better animal models since, if asbestos is an indication, it takes about three decades after initial exposure before mesothelioma begins to manifest in humans. We also need to shift away from high-dose exposure studies and begin studying "more reasonable" exposures.

FDA OVERSIGHT OF NANOTECHNOLOGY APPLICATIONS IN FOODS, FOOD PACKAGING, AND NUTRIENT DELIVERY[11]

Presenter: Laura M. Tarantino[12]

Tarantino began her talk by remarking that many of the questions asked during the first session, coupled with some of the concepts that Philbert broached, served as an excellent lead-in to the issue of regulation and the challenge of risk identification. She remarked that the focus of her presentation would be the scope of FDA's authority and oversight over foods, food ingredients, and nutrients and that she would be providing an overview of the regulatory framework currently in place.

Tarantino recommended the *FDA Nanotechnology Task Force Report*, which was issued in July 2007 as a source of information about the state of the science of biological interactions among nanomaterials (at that time—if the report were written today, its synopsis of the state of the science would be slightly different). The report also includes an analysis and recommendations for science issues and an analysis and recommendations for regulatory policy issues. Tarantino remarked that she would not be going into detail about the report but that she did want to highlight

---

[11] This section is a paraphrased summary of Tarantino's presentation.
[12] Laura M. Tarantino, PhD, is Director of the Office of Food Additive Safety in the Center for Food Safety and Applied Nutrition, FDA.

a couple of its "bottom line" messages regarding regulatory policy issues. These are issues that need to be considered soon because some of the nanomaterials mentioned and described during the previous presentations have already started appearing in food:

- Can FDA identify products containing nanoscale materials?
- What is the scope of FDA's authorities to evaluate the safety and effectiveness of such products?

One of the conclusions of the *FDA Nanotechnology Task Force Report* was that the scope of FDA's authorities depends on whether a product is subject to pre-market authorization. (The classic example of pre-market authorization is a new prescription drug, where there is a fairly rigid, robust pre-market approval process that encompasses both the product itself and the manufacturing methods. Only some types of food products are subject to a similar process.) For a product subject to premarket authorization, there is at least the presumption that FDA can demand the information (e.g., about particle size) and data (i.e., from the requisite tests) necessary to ensure that the product meets the safety standard before its approval. Tarantino remarked that this demand implies that "we know what to ask for" with respect to what kind of testing needs to be done. She said that she would be addressing only what types of products require pre-market authorization, not what kind of testing is required of those products.

The Spectrum of FDA Oversight Over Foods

FDA exercises a range of authorities over foods, with only certain types of food items requiring premarket authorization. Tarantino identified three categories of food items that she said were "somewhat arbitrary," but the categorization makes it a little easier to understand the spectrum of FDA oversight:

1. Dietary ingredients in dietary supplements
2. Colors added to food
3. Food additives and ingredients
   a. "Direct" food additives (substances that are added directly to foods [e.g., sweeteners, emulsifiers]).

b. Food contact substances (e.g., substances added to the food packaging—Tarantino referred to some of the examples mentioned during previous presentations)

c. Food ingredients whose use is generally recognized as safe (GRAS) (this category encompasses a wide spectrum of situations in terms of the kind of regulatory authorities the FDA has with respect to pre–market approval)

The first pre–market approval enacted for any food product didn't occur until the Food Additives Amendment (FAA) of the Food Drug & Cosmetic Act was enacted in 1958, requiring all manufacturers to establish safety for any new food additives. The amendment includes a very broad definition of "food additive," which as written covers everything from carrots and stew to aspartame. It established a new standard of safety; the reasonable certainty that no harm will result, and required pre–market approval for all food additives but also provided for a series of exemptions. One important exemption is GRAS. Two years later, there was another amendment to the Act, the Color Additive Amendment, which defined and required premarket approval for color additives. So while color additives are exempt from food additive regulatory policies, they have their own set of rules.

Food Contact Substances

Tarantino said that the regulatory situation with food contact substance is "probably most analogous to the new drug situation." Food contact substances include all materials that could migrate from food packaging into food, and they require a mandatory notification process and approval before marketing. Approval is restricted to the notifier and the particular notified substance; and requires FDA authorization for marketing.

Food and Color Additives

As with food contact substances, food additives (which include emulsifiers, sweeteners, etc.) and color additives also require approval before marketing. The regulation ordinarily includes identity (e.g., chemical structure, if chemical structure is an identifying feature) and levels of use (if important) and may also include requirements regarding the manufacturing process and specifications for contaminants. In short, it covers all those circumstances necessary to ensure that any manufacturer that uses the additive in compliance with regulation is using it safely. The difference between this type of regulation and regulation for food contact substances is that the former is generic. Once a regulation for a particular additive is in the books, anyone can use that product as long as they are in compliance with the regulation.

GRAS

At the other end of the FDA regulatory spectrum are food ingredients whose use is GRAS. GRAS food additives are exempt from the previously described pre-market approval process. This is a very practical and useful exemption—one based on the notion that if experts who are qualified to judge safety recognize and agree that an ingredient is safe, then there should be no need for an independent review and approval by FDA. An "expert" is somebody qualified by training or experience. He or she does not have to be a government official. What the GRAS exemption effectively means is that companies seeking to market a new food ingredient can make a determination that their use of the ingredient is GRAS, although they run the risk that the FDA will disagree. To minimize that risk, the FDA has implemented a voluntary notification process whereby manufacturers or those who wish to market a substance that they believe is GRAS can receive feedback from the FDA prior to marketing the product. While there is no pre-market approval requirement for GRAS additives, there is a burden to show that the ingredient in question meets the food additive safety standard; additionally, experts must agree that the ingredient meets that standard.

Dietary Ingredients in Dietary Supplements

Dietary ingredients in dietary supplements are exempt from the definition of food additive and do not require pre–market approval. Tarantino defined a dietary ingredient as "essentially the thing you take the dietary supplement for." Other dietary supplement additives (e.g., color additives or added sweeteners) are still regulated under the color or food additive rubric. However, "new dietary ingredients" (i.e., those that one cannot show were marketed before October 15, 1994) are subject to required notification, whereby the FDA must be notified 75 days before the product is marketed. So this is not a formal pre–market approval process, but it does give the FDA a chance to hear about the product.

Nutrients, by the way, can fall under either the dietary ingredient or food ingredient rubric, depending on whether they are added to dietary supplements (in which case they would be classified as a dietary ingredient) or food (in which case they would be classified as a food ingredient).

Where Does Nanotechnology Fall Within This Spectrum?

This wide range of regulatory authorities over food serves as a "pretty adaptable system," Tarantino said, and nano-sized product ingredients, or nanomaterials, are really just a "special case of something that we have been doing all along." Consider, for example, a food additive regulation for a particular emulsifier. The regulation would include specification for all contaminants anticipated when the regulation was written (i.e., specification for the maximum amount of contaminant allowed). If the manufacturing process for that particular emulsifier changed in such a way that the regulation still applies and yet the process produces a new, unanticipated contaminant, that would create a new problem which would need to be dealt with accordingly—that is, by doing the requisite testing. The same would be true of the use of nanotechnology or nanomaterials. The burden of proof is on the manufacturer to show that what they have done differently does not affect the safety of the product, even though there may be nothing in that particular regulation about particle size. If some sort of change has been made that may impact safety, then the change requires testing. The challenge is in the nature of the testing. As Tarantino said, "The trick here is: What questions do you ask? And how do you do that testing?" Ideally, the manufacturer should be talking with the FDA at that point and having some sort of dialogue about what type of safety data to collect and how to conduct the necessary testing. Tarantino urged, "If you've made a change that requires some testing, you really ought to be talking to us."

There are two main questions to consider when a change is made:

1. Has changing the size affected the safety? Again, if it has, then the requisite testing must be conducted.
2. Is it the same substance? If it is not, then the appropriate rules must be followed. If, for example, it has been changed in a way

that now requires pre-market approval whereas it did not before, then pre-market approval must be sought.

The burden of proof is greater with GRAS ingredients. The use of a substance in the nano form may or may not be GRAS, even if the use of substance in the macro form is GRAS. It is difficult to argue that the nanoform of a GRAS macro substance is automatically itself GRAS because not only must the manufacturer show that the nanosized substance meets the safety standard, they must also show that the information they are relying on to make that statement is generally available and recognized and related specifically to the substance under consideration (i.e., even a nanosized substance). Gathering these data may be a very difficult thing to do in this fast-evolving emerging field of nanoscience and nanotechnology.

Recent FDA Actions

The FDA participated in a recent exercise jointly sponsored by the Project on Emerging Nanotechnologies at the Woodrow Wilson International Center for Scholars and the Grocery Manufacturers Association (GMA) that involved considering three case studies of potential applications of nanotechnology in food packaging. For each case, the participants considered what kinds of testing would be necessary, what kinds of things would be considered during the approval process, and generally what the approval process would encompass. The exercise resulted in a report, *Assuring the Safety of Nanomaterials in Food Packaging: The Regulatory Process and Key Issues*, which is published on the Wilson website.[13] Tarantino said it was a very useful exercise—it was a training of sorts for FDA reviewers, and it gave developers of these types of products a chance to talk about some of the issues with both FDA and EPA regulators.

Additionally, there was an FDA-sponsored public meeting on September 8, 2008, designed to seek input on determining the data and test methods that are available and to hear public comments and concerns regarding nanomaterials in food. Tarantino reiterated that the FDA is very interested in receiving as much input as possible from people who are either thinking that they might need to conduct safety tests as they

---

[13] Available online at http://www.nanotechproject.org/publications/archive/nano_food_packaging/. Accessed January 19, 2009.

develop these types of products or already conducting such tests. Tarantino said that the comments from this meeting are currently being analyzed, and she urged workshop participants to use the meeting website as a source of information about what types of questions that FDA thinks that people ought to be considering as they move forward with developing food products with nanosized materials.

"We know that people want guidance," Tarantino said. People want and need to know what to do and how to do it when developing their products. But this is not going to be an easy thing to provide, she said, partly because nanotechnology is not a single entity. It is a new technology that encompasses many different entities, and there is no checklist for determining safety. She emphasized again that the trick is in knowing what questions to ask. Tarantino said that identifying these questions is something that could be done as a collaborative exercise between the FDA and the developer of the product. She referred to an earlier comment about the fact that much of what is going on in the area of food nanotechnology is occurring "behind closed doors." She made an appeal "to open that door at least a crack. Come on in as early as possible." She said that, on a positive note, there is a lot of knowledge and information about the materials that are being used to develop these new products. But many practical questions still remain unanswered and those are where the discussions with FDA really need to take place, for example with respect to what these materials do in the gut and what effects they may have in the context of a complex food matrix.

While there is no complete written guidance available yet, Tarantino said that the FDA has updated its guidance for food contact substances to include some language about particle size. In December 2007, two statements were added to the *Preparation for Premarket Submissions for Food Contact Substances: Chemistry Recommendations*:[14]

1. Section II.A.5. Physical/Chemical Specifications: "In cases where particle size is important to achieving the technical effect or may relate to toxicity, sponsors should describe particle size, size distribution, and morphology, as well as any size-dependent properties."
2. Section II.C. Technical Effect: "If technical effect is dependent on particle size, sponsors should present data that demonstrate

---

[14] Available online at http://www.cfsan.fda.gov/~dms/opa3pmnc.html. Accessed January 19, 2009.

the specific properties of the particles that make them useful for food-contact applications."

In conclusion, Tarantino said that the more the FDA can be engaged in dialogue with sponsors, the more likely the agency will be able to write guidance that makes sense, is helpful, and is fully protective of public health. She again encouraged early consultation with the Agency for any food or food packaging product with nanomaterial, even if "it's only a gleam in your eye." If it is something that could potentially wind up in food, "the sooner [the FDA] knows and the more we can talk, the better."

REGULATORY ISSUES CONCERNING FOOD AND NUTRIENT PRODUCTS CONTAINING NANOMATERIALS[15]

Presenter: Fred H. Degnan[16]

After some introductory remarks, including that he would be addressing much of the same territory that Tarantino covered but from a practicing lawyer perspective, Degnan identified two key regulatory issues with nanomaterials in food:

1. Whether FDA's statutory authorities provide sufficient tools to evaluate and regulate the safety of nanomaterials with novel properties when used in food, food packaging, and dietary supplements.
2. Whether FDA's existing procedures and systems are adequate to evaluate and regulate the safety of nanomaterials with novel properties when used in food, food packaging, and dietary supplements.

He emphasized the term "nanomaterials with novel properties," reiterating Tarantino's comments with respect to whether the substance in question is truly novel. The answer to the first question (above), he said, is a "resounding yes" with the possible exception of the safety system for dietary supplements which, as Tarantino alluded, is less comprehensive

---

[15] This section is a paraphrased summary of Degnan's presentation.
[16] Fred H. Degnan, JD, is a partner in King & Spalding's Washington office, where he specializes in food and drug law.

and less rigorous than the safety systems for other food items. Nonetheless, the system for supplements does provide a mechanism for evaluating the safety of those materials. The answer to the second question is, again, a "big yes" with respect to foods, food packaging, and color additives. But, again, with respect to dietary supplements, the current system is not as comprehensive, but nonetheless does exist.

Degnan argued, however, that "There is a 'but'.... These systems really do need to be augmented by [written] guidance specifically addressed to nanomaterials." While Degnan agreed with Tarantino that coming to the Agency and having discussions "would be wonderful," he said that written guidance would provide the most value for both producers, and from a transparency perspective, the public. This is true even if that guidance evolves and changes over time as more information is gathered through dialogue with sponsors and experience with the technology.

Degnan commented on the complexity of the food supply, stating that the "good news" is that the Food, Drug, and Cosmetic Act (the "FDC Act") reflects this complexity and contains a number of different "safety" standards. These standards vary according to the food itself, the use of a food substance(s), the conditions under which the food is made and held, and the ingredients or substances migrating into the food. Degnan remarked that the focus of his presentation would be on the last issue: ingredients and migrants; that is, the migration of substances from packaging into food.

He explained that, as Tarantino alluded, the critical difference in rigor that accompanies the different safety standards in the FDC Act depends in large part upon whether pre–market approval requirements or post-market enforcement authorities apply. The FDA has not always had a pre–market authority system in place. For the first 60 years of federal regulation, FDA's only authority over food was based on post-market enforcement constructs, whereby the Agency had to go out and find food safety problems and then convince the courts that the problems rendered the food unlawful. In 1958, with enactment of the Food Additives Amendment (FAA), Congress enacted a pre–market approval system, whereby companies were required to have ingredients meeting the definition of "food additive" approved by the FDA before being able to lawfully market the ingredients. The FAA shifted the burden of proving safety from FDA to industry, creating a huge difference between the post-market and pre-market approval schemes. Of the more than 120 amendments to the FDC Act, the FAA is among "the best" in Degnan's view. He characterized it as a "remarkably good piece of legislation," one that is still vibrant and relevant today.

Remarkably, the safety issues presented by the use of nanomaterials with novel properties in food are almost identical to those that presented 50 years ago and which led to the passage of the FAA. These issues presented themselves then largely because of the technological and chemistry developments related to World War II. Synthetic food ingredients were being manufactured very suddenly, and the FDA was confronted with literally thousands of new ingredients whose safety had never been reviewed. The FAA was designed to address a public health scenario with the following:

- Potentially thousands of novel substances to be added to food
- Only a few such substances specifically tested/reviewed for safety
- An existing regulatory system hampered by limited resources
- Public/private sector concerns about under/over regulation

What makes the FAA so vibrant and effective? Degnan noted that the objectives of the FAA are actually twofold: (1) to assure safety and (2) to foster innovation in food technology. Degnan identified three tools that have made it possible to accomplish these dual objectives:

1. Pre–market clearance with burden of proof on the sponsor.
2. A rigorous but non-absolute safety standard (i.e., "reasonable certainty of no harm"). The FAA contains only one absolute binding standard: the Delaney Clause. (The Delaney Clause effectively states that no additive could be deemed safe or given FDA approval if found to cause cancer in humans or experimental animals.) Other than that, as Degnan stated, the statute requires a food additive to be "safe" but does not define in any meaningful way a standard for assessing an additive is "safe."
3. A broad, comprehensive definition of "food additive" coupled with reasonable expectations, including one flexible, forward-looking exception for substances Generally Recognized as Safe (GRAS).

The GRAS Exemption

A food additive is defined, in part, as "any substance that directly or indirectly may reasonably become a component of food." This is a very broad definition and one that led Congress to apply certain exceptions. Pesticide chemical residues, for example, are not considered food additives and instead are regulated under another (nonfood) rubric. The most important exception, however, is for GRAS substances—that is, substances that are generally recognized as safe by qualified experts on the basis of knowledge derived from scientific procedures. Degnan characterized the GRAS concept as "the grease, … the element that allows the FAA to work, and it's been that way since the inception of FDA's regulation of food additives in 1958." The GRAS provision allows the FDA to prioritize its limited resources and examine only those new and novel substances that demand its attention. And, it provides a flexible way to address food safety concerns in an efficient manner.

Degnan briefly described two recent important applications of the GRAS concept: (1) The GRAS provision was critical to the Agency's ability to implement its transgenic plant policy. The provision allowed FDA to treat as GRAS most transferred genetic materials (primarily nucleic acids) thereby avoiding time-consuming food additive approval and unnecessary restraints on innovative technology. (2) More recent is FDA's reliance on a voluntary notification process that offers a prompt and thorough review and encourages industry submissions. Under the process industry collects publicly available data with respect to the safety of a given use and assembles a panel of experts to review the information and opine on the safety of the subject compound for a use or set of uses. FDA, in turn, relies on the assembled data and the expert opinions to evaluate whether a question with respect to GRAS status is presented.

Degnan emphasized that determining that a substance is GRAS is "not a shortcut or loophole." He said, "It is far from it. In my view, making a GRAS determination is harder than making a safety determination, because to be GRAS a substance has to have all of the fundamental proof that would accompany a food additive, *and* that proof must be publicly available. It's a demanding standard."

Nanomaterials with Novel Properties and GRAS

One of the key regulatory questions with respect to nanomaterials with novel properties is whether they can be considered GRAS. Or, because of the practical difficulty involved in establishing general recognition of a novel substance, is it an oxymoron or contradiction to say "GRAS nanomaterials with novel properties?" This is a key issue currently in consideration at the FDA and one that Tarantino and her colleagues must consider in the context of what was done with transgenic plants and, in 1997, with the notification policy. Degnan noted that the issue also relates to a question that Groth asked earlier: Can a line be drawn in the spectrum of differently sized materials such that those materials that fall on one side can be considered GRAS?

Degnan remarked that the situation is different with dietary supplements. As Tarantino had stated earlier, dietary ingredients in dietary supplements qualify as an exemption to the definition of a "food additive," and thus are not subject to a pre–market approval process. The regulation process for dietary supplements is a post–market approval process, and the only way the FDA can take a dietary supplement off the market is to show that the supplement presents a "significant or unreasonable risk of illness or injury." This is a difficult burden of proof for FDA to meet. However, there is a pre-market "notification" requirement for certain dietary ingredients. All dietary ingredients not used in dietary supplements before October 15, 1994, are considered "New Dietary Ingredients" (NDIs) and, as such, must be the subject of a pre-market notification filed with FDA 75 days before marketing. The notification must contain the basis for the manufacturer's conclusion that a supplement containing an NDI is "reasonably expected to be safe." Failure to provide that information gives the FDA reason to argue in enforcement action (i.e., post-market action) that an inadequate basis exists to determine whether the general adulteration standard is met. While not the most efficient system, it does provide FDA with a mechanism for evaluating a new ingredient, including a nanomaterial with novel properties.

Degnan noted a potential complication arises because some substances can be classified as either "food additives" or dietary ingredients, depending on how they are used. Vitamin D added to orange juice, for example, is considered a food additive and is regulated accordingly. On the other hand, vitamin D as an ingredient in a dietary supplement is considered a dietary ingredient and thereby falls under a different regulatory rubric. This variation in how nutrients are regulated, depending on how they are used in or added to foods, "could well in time prove to be another significant regulatory issue."

So for dietary ingredients in dietary supplements, the issues are the following:

- What criteria will FDA apply for determining whether nanomaterials with novel properties are "new dietary ingredients"? Degnan noted that presumably an effort would be made to use the same criteria used for evaluating the safety of a food additive.
- What criteria will FDA apply in the "notification" process for evaluating safety of dietary ingredients nanomaterials with novel properties?

For other food substances (i.e., food and color additives and GRAS nanomaterials), the issues are the following:

- What criteria will FDA apply for evaluating the safety of nanomaterials? Specifically, what are the criteria for (1) substances already holding approved additive status, including both food and color additives; (2) substances already under consideration by regulation or the notification process as GRAS; and (3) nanomaterials for use in new or unapproved substances?
- Are there circumstances under which nanomaterials will not be considered to present a safety concern? Degnan identified this issue as "the more driving question." If the answer is yes, then what factors need to be addressed to reach such a conclusion?
- Similarly, what criteria will FDA consider applicable for establishing the GRAS status of nanomaterial substances with novel properties?

Concluding Remarks

In conclusion, Degnan reiterated four points:

1. FDA's statutory pre–market authorities provide a comprehensive regulatory framework for assuring the safety of nanomaterials with novel properties for use in food and food packaging. The framework for dietary supplements is not as comprehensive but still provides a mechanism for evaluation by the agency.
2. FDA should author guidances with respect to the criteria to be followed in evaluating the safety of food, food packaging, and

supplement uses of nanomaterials with novel properties. This is key Degnan said, not only from a public confidence perspective but also from the perspective of industry. Industry needs to have in hand written guidance on the agency's criteria for showing the safety of nanomaterials of novel properties.

3. FDA should provide leadership, on both the domestic and international fronts, not only in developing guidance but in refining guidance as knowledge evolves. Degnan remarked that FDA is providing this leadership, as evident for example by Tarantino's encouragement to industry to engage in dialogue with the agency.

4. Industry must conduct research and investigations to substantiate the propriety of the use in food of nanomaterials with novel properties. While FDA needs to take a leadership role, the ultimate responsibility is still always going to fall on industry.

As a "postscript" to the topic of FDA's regulation of nanotechnology in the context of food and dietary ingredients, Degnan facetiously commented that the Food, Drug, and Cosmetic Act is "misbranded," in light of the fact that the Act provides FDA authority to regulate far more than just food, drugs, and cosmetics. His point: "There is a whole universe of products that FDA regulates and each type of product (i.e., drugs, medical devices, cosmetics, etc.) is subject to advancement with nanomaterials with novel properties." The potentially broad use of nanomaterials with novel properties in FDA regulated products is another reason why the FDA should provide leadership and why there needs to be discussion among the various agency centers involved with developments and ideas concerning nanomaterials and their safety. There are also potential concerns about exposure to nanomaterials from a worker, or Occupational Safety and Health Administration (OSHA) perspective. Finally, Degnan commented that the FDA could also provide leadership on the international front, where current regulatory approaches range from laissez-faire to moratoria on research involving nanomaterials. The basis for providing that leadership role, Degnan reiterated, is written guidance.

OPEN DISCUSSION[17]

The second session ended with a 15-minute question and answer period. Most of the questions revolved around the issue of toxicology and testing of nanomaterials. Other topics of discussion included how to encourage early industry consultation with the FDA (and other regulatory agencies); when to expect written guidance on nanomaterials in food from the FDA; and the difference between foods with targeted delivery capacities and drugs.

Toxicology and Testing of Nanomaterials

Doyle opened the discussion by commenting on Philbert's "very intriguing" comments about how scientists can apply what they already know about physical properties (from having studied other substances, such as asbestos fibers) to nanomaterials. He then asked if there has been any attempt by toxicologists or others to put together some sort of list of the types of things that need to be avoided when developing nanotechnology related materials. Philbert replied, "There have been various attempts." The problem, however, is that there are very little comprehensive data available. For example, there are very few published pharmacokinetic studies of nanomaterials. The difficulty lies in not knowing where the nanomaterial ends; it depends on its physical or chemical characteristics. "I think there's a lot of hand-waving going on. We need more data."

Doyle then asked if this lack of data has any bearing on activity in the area of regulatory approval and whether there won't be much regulatory activity until there are more data. Philbert replied, "We in some sense are jumping the gun because we simply don't know what we're regulating." Importantly, however, we are "laying the landscape," so that when the data do emerge, there is some context for interpreting it.

An unidentified workshop attendee remarked that the FDA is at a point where it can only examine each case individually. While doing so, the agency is building the very database in question—one that will allow the Agency to make some generalizations in the future. But it is too soon to be making those generalizations now.

---

[17] This section paraphrases the open discussion that took place at the end of the second session.

This remark was followed by a question about Degnan's emphasis on regulatory policies around "nanomaterials with novel properties" and whether the notion of novel properties included those that were unintended or unrecognized. Degnan responded by saying that intent in that context is irrelevant. The overriding intent, he said, is the ingredient or the nanomaterial itself, that is, the nanomaterial *intended* to be a component of food. He said that as long as that is the case, his remarks apply.

Workshop attendee Richard Bruner, WIL Research Laboratories, LLC, Ashland, OH, mentioned his background in preclinical animal testing of new drugs and commented on how he had attended this workshop hoping that the panelists would "lay out a platform of animal testing that we could all take back to our laboratories." He said, "Obviously that's a daunting task and is not about to happen." He remarked that animal testing is very expensive and that testing even a single nanoparticle in a typical animal profile could exhaust a small company's entire resources. He suggested that perhaps the "nanotechnology network" join forces and create an organization, much like the Chemistry Industry Institute of Toxicology (CIIT) was formed years ago, which would serve as an interface with the FDA and a filtering mechanism for all the small companies who have a need for testing requirements. The group would be a global network of toxicologists, engineers, and other scientists, and it would serve as a source of advice for the FDA and, in turn, a source of information for the scientific community about how the FDA views nanotechnology. It would also interface with regulatory agencies in other countries. "Is the pill too large to swallow?" Bruner asked.

Degnan responded, "No." He pointed to work sponsored by the International Life Sciences Institute in the late 1980s and early 1990s on transgenic food safety and conducted by an organization called the International Food Biotechnology Council (IFBC). The IFBC assembled an international array of experts who worked together for a year and a half to produce a template document addressing every aspect of safety through regulatory approval and then circulated the template worldwide for comments. The end product provided a very helpful predicate for and actually prompted FDA to develop its own guidance on transgenic crops (in May 1992). So that approach is one that makes a great deal of sense.

Philbert mentioned that the Environmental Defense Fund and DuPont have worked together to develop a set of toxicology tests for use with a wide variety of nanomaterials. However, the set of tests is still "quite expensive" and does not obviate the cost issue, but it does provide a "happy intermediate" in the sense that the toxicity tests have been shown to be very useful for ruling out formulations that are not going to work and are therefore not worth developing further. Bruner remarked that these tests run the risk, however, of being rejected by the FDA. Philbert replied that the idea is to "cherry pick" among tests as a precursor to a Good Laboratory Practice (GLP) study. He said, "I think the days of developing a chemical and then looking at the toxicity are over" and that "involving the toxicologists and the biologists from the outset is the only way to do this." Tarantino added that toxicologists and biologists from the FDA should be involved from the outset. She reiterated, "Come in before you do all the studies and talk to us, rather than at the end, and we'll be less likely to reject them."

Early Consultation with the FDA

Tarantino's last comment prompted workshop attendee Bill Jordan of the U.S. Environmental Protection Agency (EPA) to remark that the EPA regulates pesticide products that may contain nanomaterials and, like the FDA, encourages folks who are making those products to engage in dialogue with the EPA in preparation for pre-market review. Based on some of the information presented at this workshop, he observed, "It would seem that there are a lot more folks who should have been doing that than actually have." Jordan asked if this might also be the case with the FDA. He then asked what regulatory agencies, trade associations, or other organizations can do to encourage people who are developing these technologies to communicate more freely and earlier with the regulatory bodies that have responsibility over those products.

Tarantino replied that there have been a few applications and a number of what the FDA calls "pre-submission consultations," meaning consultations conducted before formal submissions. She would not be surprised if there were some products out there for which manufacturers probably should have approached the FDA but did not. Although again (as Philbert elaborated during his presentation), things labeled "nano" may or may not actually involve nanotechnology or nanomaterials. Tarantino said that she didn't know how the FDA could encourage earlier consultations. She noted the early and frequent consultations sought by industry when transgenic plants emerged as a regulatory issue, which was very helpful for the FDA. Degnan added that there were a number of factors that motivated the transgenic plant industry's cooperation and consultation, a large one being consumer acceptance.

Timeline for FDA Guidance

An unidentified workshop attendee asked Tarantino if the FDA knows approximately when it will issue guidance on the topics that Degnan addressed during his presentation and when interim guidances will be available. Tarantino said that she could not provide a date but emphasized that the FDA recognizes the utility of such guidance, particularly with respect to food additives (which is where her office is most involved). With respect to interim guidances, those are done in a "cyclic manner." She said to expect updates for some of the other guidances (i.e., in addition to the already completed updated guidance for food contact substances) "in the next year or so."

When Does a Food Become a Drug?

Workshop attendee Van Hubbard, NIH, commented that nanotechnology has the ability to target specific tissues. But as scientists begin targeting tissues, where is the point at which this targeting becomes a pharmaceutical delivery? Degnan said that there was a legal response to the question and that the answer hinges on intent: "Foods can tout their effects on the structure and function of the body and do that lawfully. As soon as, however, a food even implies some therapeutic effect—some effect to treat, to mitigate, to cure, prevent or even diagnose disease— … it becomes a drug." When it becomes a drug, a much more demanding and possibly clearer set of requirements with respect to the testing of both safety and effectiveness come into play. Whether targeted delivery makes something a food or drug depends on intent of the manufacturer, which can be implied and inferred by FDA.

Philbert commented on the emergence of Internet communities with their own sense of what foods can do: Manufacturers can now introduce components into their foods knowing that those components (and any implied therapeutic effects) will be discussed in the blogosphere, thereby circumventing the FDA process. He asked if there was any way that the FDA could regulate this type of activity. Tarantino said that part of the answer depends on whether these foods are being advertised as dietary supplements and whether the FDA can take action; and another part depends on what sort of claims are being made and whether those claims are supported (i.e., if not, then the FDA can take action). She referred to Hubbard's original question and said that, in many cases, the line is blurred and will probably become even more blurred in the future as nanomaterials become very effective nutrient delivery vehicles. Degnan pointed out however, that nutrient delivery is in fact a perfectly appropriate food and dietary supplement use. A manufacturer can lawfully make claims about nutrients, and there is a rubric for dealing with those claims. Only if that nutrient delivery is used for a therapeutic purpose does one enter "drug territory."

4

Educating and Informing Consumers About Applications of Nanotechnology to Food Products

This chapter summarizes the presentations and discussions that occurred during the third and final session of the workshop. The first presenter, Julia Moore of the Woodrow Wilson International Center for Scholars, used polling data and results from four years of focus group work to argue that public opinion about nanotechnology being applied in the food industry is essentially "up for grabs." A large majority of Americans know little about nanotechnology and have yet to form an opinion about its use. She identified several key lessons learned from past "ag-biotech" experience about public engagement with new technologies.

The second presenter, Carl Batt of Cornell University, spent most of his time describing how he and his collaborators designed the *Too Small to See: Zoom into Nanotechnology* museum exhibition. He discussed the challenges faced when trying to communicate ideas about size and scale to the public and how *Too Small to See* overcomes some of these challenges. He briefly described production of *Nanooze*, a nanoscience magazine for children that is available in print and online.

The third and final presenter of the session, Jean Halloran of Consumers Union, provided consumer perspective insights and responses to several of the ideas and issues that other workshop presenters and attendees had raised up until that point. She commented on the difference between knowing about a technology and accepting that technology; gaps in knowledge about the safety of nanotechnologies in food; consumers' fear of the unknown, particularly in foods; the importance of regulation and how consumers need to know that they are being protected; and the importance of consumer choice.

The session ended with a lengthy panel discussion with all 10 presenters of the day participating on the panel. Most of the questions and comments revolved around issues related to consumer behavior and public engagement, although the issue of regulatory uncertainty re-emerged as well.

NANOTECHNOLOGY AND FOOD: THE PUBLIC KNOWS "NANO"[1]

Presenter: Julia A. Moore[2]

Moore began her talk by remarking that the public knows very little about nanotechnology in food. Within her organization, the Woodrow Wilson International Center for Scholars, the Project on Emerging Nanotechnologies, has probably done more focus group and public opinion polling on public attitudes and perceptions, as well as how to influence those attitudes and perceptions, than any other organization. That said, it was actually the National Science Foundation (NSF) that supported the first public opinion polls on nanotechnology in 2004. One of the questions posed in that initial NSF poll was: How much have you heard about nanotechnology? The question was posed again in a 2008 study conducted by Peter D. Hart Research Associates (on behalf of the Project on Emerging Nanotechnologies), and the numbers were basically the same (Moore presented the 2008 data, which involved surveying 1,003 adults nationwide[3]):

- 49 percent replied that they had "heard nothing at all";
- 26 percent said they had "heard just a little";
- 17 percent had "heard some";
- 7 percent had "heard a lot"; and
- 1 percent were "unsure."

Moore remarked that most of the 17 percent who said that they "heard some" probably in fact knew nothing about nanotechnology. She said that it is easy to imagine somebody getting a phone call and being told,

---

[1] This section is a paraphrased summary of Julia Moore's presentation.
[2] Julia A. Moore is Deputy Director of the Project on Emerging Nanotechnologies, an initiative of the Woodrow Wilson International Center for Scholars & The Pew Charitable Trusts.
[3] SOURCE: Peter D. Hart Research, Inc. 2008. "Awareness of and Attitudes Toward Nano- technology and Federal Regulatory Agencies." Available online at http://www. pewtrusts.org/our_work_report_detail.aspx?id=30539. Accessed January 26, 2009.

"Hey, I'm going to talk to you about nanotechnology …" and the person saying, "Yeah, I've heard something about nano.…"

According to the same 2008 poll, when asked what their initial impressions were about the benefits and risks of nanotechnology (i.e., whether the benefits will outweigh the risks or vice versa), many people were unsure:

- 48 percent replied "not sure";
- 25 percent replied "the benefits and risks will be about equal";
- 20 percent replied "benefits will outweigh risks"; and
- 7 percent replied "risks will outweigh benefits."

Although, as shown in Figure 4-1, the percentage of people that were unsure decreases as familiarity with nanotechnology increases (i.e., 65 percent of people who had "heard nothing" were "not sure" about the benefits and risks, whereas only 10 percent of those had heard "a lot" said that they were "not sure").

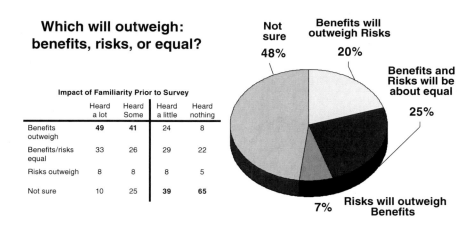

Which will outweigh: benefits, risks, or equal?

Impact of Familiarity Prior to Survey

	Heard a lot	Heard Some	Heard a little	Heard nothing
Benefits outweigh	49	41	24	8
Benefits/risks equal	33	26	29	22
Risks outweigh	8	8	8	5
Not sure	10	25	39	65

Not sure 48%
Benefits will outweigh Risks 20%
Benefits and Risks will be about equal 25%
Risks will outweigh Benefits 7%

FIGURE 4-1 How people perceive the risks and benefits of nanotechnology without being told anything about nanotechnology prior to being surveyed. The table on the lower left breaks the responses down according to how familiar with nanotechnology respondents said they were prior to the survey. Image courtesy of Peter D. Hart Research Associates, Inc., on behalf of the Project on Emerging Technologies.

When people were provided with some information about nanotechnology prior to the survey (i.e., the pollster read some sentences about what nanotechnology and its applications are), the percentage of people who were unsure dropped from 48 to 9 percent (see Figure 4-2):

- 38 percent replied "benefits and risks will be about equal";
- 30 percent replied "benefits will outweigh risks";
- 23 percent replied "risks will outweigh benefits"; and
- 9 percent replied "not sure."

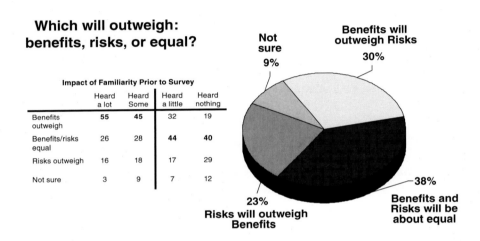

Which will outweigh: benefits, risks, or equal?

Impact of Familiarity Prior to Survey

	Heard a lot	Heard Some	Heard a little	Heard nothing
Benefits outweigh	55	45	32	19
Benefits/risks equal	26	28	44	40
Risks outweigh	16	18	17	29
Not sure	3	9	7	12

FIGURE 4-2 How people perceive the risks and benefits of nanotechnology after being informed about the potential risks and benefits of nanotechnology. The table on the lower left breaks the responses down according to how familiar with nanotechnology respondents said they were prior to the survey. Image courtesy of Peter D. Hart Research Associates, Inc., on behalf of the Project on Emerging Nanotechnologies.

The take-home message from these survey data, Moore said, is that "public opinion is really up for grabs when it comes to nanotechnology. The public really doesn't know very much to have an opinion."

When asked about the benefits that they would like to see derived from nanotechnology, indeed from any new technology, Americans consider the potential medical applications to be the most important (e.g., "a cure for cancer"). More specifically, in a 2006 study, surveyed members of the U.S. public identified the following as the most important potential benefits of nanotechnology[4]:

- Medical applications (31 percent)
- Better consumer products (27 percent)
- General progress, better life (12 percent)
- Environmental protection (8 percent)
- Food and nutrition (6 percent)
- Economy, jobs (4 percent)

Moore remarked that, interestingly, when the same question is asked in Europe, respondents generally indicate that they are much more concerned with environmental issues (e.g., environmental clean-up methods) than U.S. residents are. Of note, only 6 percent of respondents indicated that "food and nutrition" benefits are one of the most important potential benefits of nanotechnology. This is consistent with most other new technologies. While people are generally delighted to have new technologies put to use in computers, telephones, etc., even tennis racquets, the idea of having a new technology applied to a food is often viewed as "yucky." That is something to keep in mind, Moore said, when considering or trying to project what public perceptions of this new technology (i.e., nanotechnology) will be.

While one might expect most people to learn about nanotechnology in the classroom, through government education programs, or from science societies, such as the National Academy of Sciences, Moore said that this is not the case. Most people learn about nanotechnology in grocery, clothing, and drug stores. Moore encouraged workshop attendees to visit http://www.nanotechproject.org/inventories/consumer and browse the 800+ consumer products, particularly products in the "food and beverage" category that are self-identified as "nano" or nanotechnology-based. As Philbert had remarked earlier, being self-identified as nano does not mean that a product is in fact nanotechnology based. It means only that the manufacturer is making that claim.

In addition to the fact that only a small percentage of people identify food and beverage benefits as an important potential benefit of nanotechnology, Moore said "another piece of bad news" is that many people are

---

[4] J Macoubried. 2006. Nanotechnology: Public concerns, reasoning and trust in government. *Public Understanding of Science* 15:221-241.

worried about the overall safety of the U.S. food supply. When asked how the food supply has changed over the last five years (as part of the same 2008 survey cited previously):

- 39 percent replied that it "has become somewhat less safe";
- 22 percent replied that it "has become much less safe";
- 22 percent replied that it "has become somewhat more safe";
- 7 percent replied that it "has become much more safe";
- 6 percent replied that it "has been unchanged"; and
- 4 percent replied that they were "not sure."

Moore emphasized that even though these responses reflect perceptions, not necessarily reality, the results are consistent with other polling data. This concern about safety raises the question, who does the American public trust, and where does it place its confidence with respect to maximizing the benefits and minimizing the risks of scientific and technological advancements? Other polling data show that the public trusts the U.S. government (i.e., the USDA, FDA, and EPA), independent scientists, and independent agencies much more than they trust businesses and companies. Basically, Moore said, the public wants to know that the FDA is taking care of the safety of the food supply.

Moore emphasized that the public is not averse to nanotechnology. For example, according to the same survey data collected by Peter D. Hart Research Associates, Inc. (on behalf of the Project on Emerging Nanotechnologies), when asked if they would use food storage products enhanced with nanotechnology, 12 percent said yes, 73 percent said that they need more information about the health risks and benefits, and 13 percent said no. When asked if they would purchase food enhanced with nanotechnology, 7 percent said yes, 62 percent said that they need more information about the health risks and benefits, and 29 percent said no. But they do need more information.

In summary:

- A large majority of Americans still have heard little or nothing about nanotechnology.
- A large portion of the public does not have an opinion on the trade-offs between the risks and benefits of nanotechnology.
- The U.S. public is more comfortable with government or independent oversight than industry self-regulation of new technologies. Moore noted that this is an important point to

consider because the U.S. public relies on industry to provide safe products (i.e., because too much regulation would stifle innovation).

- The current lack of awareness presents an opportunity for the government and industry to establish confidence in nanotechnology. Moore said that if those involved in the food sector think that nanotechnology is going to provide strong benefits for consumers, then they really need to get out there and start shaping that still unformed perception of nanotechnology.
- The U.S. public values nanotechnology medical benefits over food and nutrition. Moore remarked that a single highly beneficial application of nanotechnology, not necessarily in food but more likely in medicine, would cause people to "immediately identify" with nanotechonology.

Moore listed four lessons to be learned from the "ag-biotech experience":

1. Build public trust in a strong, credible U.S. and international oversight process. The American public is much more likely to accept a new technology if they think someone is looking after their interest. If they don't think that anyone is looking after their interest, they will reject the new technology.
2. Make sure nanotechnology's environmental and health benefits and safety are confirmed by independent research.
3. Demonstrate concern for consumer choice and provide good consumer information. Focus group and polling studies have shown that consumers like choice. For example, people do not like being told that they have to use sunscreen with nanotechnology and that they don't really have a choice. Consumers become upset when they find out that a product that they have been using all along has nanotechnology in it without their knowledge (i.e., there is no mention of nanomaterials in the labeling). In order to build confidence in a new technology, it is important to provide consumers with information and to make sure that they have a choice about whether to use the new technology or not. This is true even though people do not necessarily actually look at the information. But they want somebody to have the information. They want it to be transparent and available.

4. Offer opportunities for public input into the technology's development and regulation. A key issue with respect to engaging the public is that the engagement does not involve just telling people that nanotechnology is "all about controlling matter on a 1–100 nm scale." That is not the type of communication they want. Focus group studies have shown that people want to have input into whether or not the new technology is going to be used in ways that they think are important, and they want to feel that they are being heard.

Moore concluded by encouraging people to visit the Project on Emerging Nanotechnologies website, where more information on the focus group and polling studies that she discussed is posted: http://www.nanotechproject.org. Moore also provided a hand-out for workshop attendees that contained some of the same data she presented.[5]

CHALLENGES IN EDUCATING CONSUMERS ABOUT EMERGING TECHNOLOGIES[6]

Presenter: Carl Batt[7]

Batt began with a few comments about his scientific research on biodegradable plastics. His research team has developed a process that involves coupling a particular enzyme to a magnetic bead and growing large masses of bacterial polyester. The polymer masses stay in place *in situ* and are being used for cancer therapy and other therapeutic applications. Batt and his students are also doing what Batt refers to as "nanostructured prospecting," or "reverse food science," and they are investigating the use of chemically modified particles in pesticide detection.

But the focus of his talk was not his scientific research, rather his participation in development of *Too Small to See: Zoom into Nanotechnology*, a 5,000-square foot traveling museum exhibition supported by

---

[5] Awareness of and Attitudes Toward Nanotechnology and Federal Regulatory Agencies: A Report of Findings, available online at http://www.pewtrusts.org/uploadedFiles/www.pewtrustsorg/Reports/Nanotechnologies/Hart_NanoPoll_2007.pdf. Accessed February 11, 2009.

[6] This section is a paraphrased summary of Carl Batt's presentation.

[7] Carl A. Batt, PhD, is Liberty Hyde Bailey Professor of Food Science and co-founder and former director of the Nanobiotechnology Center, Cornell University, Ithaca, NY.

the NSF, and the magazine *Nanooze*. Batt remarked that, for the remainder of his presentation, while describing these two programs, he would try to convey what he and his colleagues think are the "underlying foundations" of what people know and how they think about size and scale.

Too Small to See

When Batt and his colleagues began developing *Too Small to See*, rather than trying to get a sense of what the public knows about nanotechnology, which is essentially nothing, they formulated a set of questions designed to get a sense of what people know and how they think about size and scale. Initially, they did ask, "Have you heard of nano?" The responses, Batt said, were based largely on the fact that people would get kind of embarrassed if they had not heard of it, and so they'd say, "yeah, yeah, I've heard of it." Slightly less than 30 percent (in the 18–22-year-old age range) to more than 70 percent (in the <8 years old age range) of respondents said that they had heard of nano. But when probed further and asked "What is nano?" most people referred to the iPod nano (or "that iPod thing"), an answer Batt said was "sort of meaningless." So Batt and his team changed the focus of the questioning. Instead, they asked people, "What is the smallest thing that you can see?" But the answers were often dependent on the respondents' environments. If someone saw a bug crawling, that would be the answer. Or if they had crumbs all over them, that would be the answer. So again, the answers were sort of meaningless. Instead, as their first line of questioning in their effort to find out what people know about size and scale and how they know it, they asked, "What is the smallest thing that you can think of?"

The answers, Batt said, were interesting. Some people identified a visible organism, like a bug, as the smallest thing they could think of; others identified something cellular as the smallest thing they could think of; and then there were people who identified either something atomic or something subatomic, like a quark or proton, as the smallest thing they could think of. Batt referred to people in one of the latter two groups as "post-atomic." The answer to this question allowed the researchers to define populations of people who thought on a macroscopic vs. microscopic vs. nanoscopic scale. The exhibitors developed a scoring system to measure people's thinking about scale, with post-atomic people earning higher "think scores." Specifically, people that identified a visible organism as the smallest thing they could think of were assigned a score of 1; people that identified something cellular were assigned a score of 2; people that identified something atomic received a 3; and people that identified something subatomic received a 4. The highest scores were among teenagers (age 16–18; see Figure 4-3). Generally, only a small fraction of people actually thinks about things "on a nanoscale world."

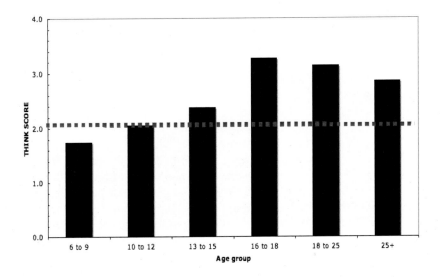

FIGURE 4-3 The range of "think scores," by age, when respondents were asked to identify the smallest thing they could think of. A higher score indicates more "sub-atomic," or nanoscopic, thinking. See text for more details.
SOURCE: Reprinted from Springer, *Journal of Nanoparticle Research,* Volume 10, Issue 7, 2008, pp. 1141-1148, Numbers, scale and symbols: the public understanding of nanotechnology, CA Batt, AM Waldron, N Broadwater, adapted from Figure 1, Copyright © (2008), with kind permission from Springer Science and Business Media.

The finding that only a small percentage of people actually think about things on a nanoscale level, combined with the reality that the average visitor to a science museum spends less than one minute in front of any individual exhibit, became the basis for *Too Small to See.* The challenge was to distill all of the information that Batt and his team wanted to convey into something that could be communicated in less than a minute (or, as Batt noted, 60,000,000,000 nanoseconds). In order to do that, they developed what they termed the "Four Concepts," or "Carl's Commandments":

- All things are made of atoms.
- Molecules have size and shape.
- At the nanometer scale, atoms are in constant motion.
- Molecules in their nanometer scale environment have unexpected properties.

Batt said the fourth point—that unexpected things happen—is what makes nanotechnology so interesting. The exhibitors decided that they wanted to hammer these four concepts at every opportunity. The four concepts also serve as a basis for every issue of *Nanooze*.

Scale and Perspective

Before describing the Four Concepts in more detail, Batt discussed how difficult it is for people to understand the concept of scale. It is hard enough to imagine a billion of something, let alone one billionth of something. Also, people have a difficult time with numbers, often interpreting "billion" and "1,000,000,000" differently. As an example, Batt referred to the widespread email scam whereby somebody claiming to be from Nigeria informs the recipient that "the sum of $1,000,000,000 USD (One Million Dollars Only)" awaits him or her. $1,000,000,000 is not a million dollars—it's a billion dollars. So figuring out 10^9 is hard, 10^{-9} even harder. Thinking small is difficult, and many people, "including probably all of us," Batt said, "can't think on those terms." Physicist Richard Feynman developed a helpful analogy: if an atom were the size of an apple, then an apple would be the size of the earth. Still, even that analogy would be difficult for most people to interpret while walking through a science exhibit.

In *Too Small to See*, everything is 100,000,000 (one hundred million) times larger than it actually is. So atoms, for example, are represented as objects that are 100,000,000 times larger than actual atoms are. Batt said that many people might wonder, "Why one hundred million? Why not a million?" As it turns out, objects smaller than 1.3 inches are considered choking hazards and cannot be included. And if the scale had been made larger, then the atoms would have been very large. A human hair at 100,000,000-fold, for example, would be the width of a river. Even at

100,000,000-fold, people have a difficult time. For example, when told what a golf ball would look like when enlarged 100,000,000 times and then asked what a pinhead would look like when enlarged to the same extent, less than 20 percent of people with lower "think scores" (i.e., below 3) answered correctly when given a choice of answers separated by two orders of magnitude. About 25 percent of people with think scores of 3 and 60 percent of people with think scores of 4 answered correctly.

In addition to their difficulty with scale, many people also have a difficult time with perspective. For example, Batt showed an image of two spheres, one in the foreground and one in the background; although the spheres are the same size, the one in the background looks larger (see Figure 4-4). When designing *Too Small to See*, the exhibitors tried to avoid these problems with scale and perspective.

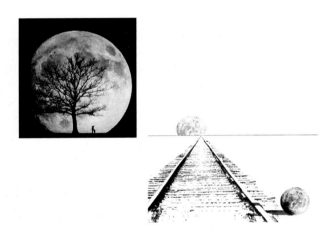

FIGURE 4-4 Images depicting the types of scale and perspective problems that the creators of *Too Small to See* tried to avoid when developing their exhibition. In the image on the right, even though the spheres are the same size, many people think that the sphere in the background is larger. In the image on the left, the orders of magnitude difference in size between the moon in the background and the tree in the foreground is not immediately apparent.
SOURCE: With permission from Carol Batt. available online at http://www.moillusions.com/2008/12/moon-optical-illusion.html. Accessed March 24, 2009.

The Four Concepts

Batt described in more detail how the museum exhibit was built around the four concepts, based on interviews conducted at the New York State Fair:

1. All things are made of atoms. The researchers asked interviewees to draw an atom, a molecule, and a piece of DNA. Interestingly, Batt said, when people tended to get DNA right, they drew the iconic double-stranded helix. Yet, they couldn't identify any of the atoms on the double helix. Most people, when they drew molecules, drew ball-and-stick figures. When drawing atoms, most people drew the Bohr model. And then there were the children that drew things that looked nothing like an atom, molecule, or piece of DNA (see Figure 4-5). The exhibitors decided that since most people that could associate with the post-atomic, or nanoscale world, did so through use of the iconic ball-and-stick image, they would use the ball-and-stick model in the exhibit. They also tried to use iconic coloration of the balls and sticks as much as possible. So when people walk into the exhibit, every time they see a ball, they recognize that ball as an atom. And again, every atom, including every digital representation, is enlarged 100,000,000 times.

2. Molecules have size and shape. The scientists showed interviewees images of a ball-and-stick model, a space-filling model, and a domain model of a molecule and then asked the interviewees to identify components of each model (see Figure 4-6). Again, people were able to identify atoms in the ball-and-stick model and, to a lesser extent, bonds in the same model. The highest "think score" was among the 13–15 years old age group, where more than 70 percent of those surveyed correctly identified atoms in the ball-and-stick model. Many people identified the domain model image as "moldy popcorn."

3. At the nanometer scale, molecules are in constant motion. This is a very important concept and one that is also very difficult to portray. With the help of artist Zack Simpson, Austin, Texas, the exhibitors developed an animated display where museum visitors could reach out and, on a screen, fold and stretch molecules (see Figure 4-7).

4. Molecules in their nanometer scale environment have unexpected properties. The greatest challenge in developing this ex-

hibit was in designing a way to show these unexpected properties, since nanoscale phenomena do not scale up. For example, the scientists built a prototype exhibit using neodymium supermagnet spheres (available online at http://www.amasci.com/amateur/beads.html), but too many visitors walked away thinking that atoms are like little magnets.

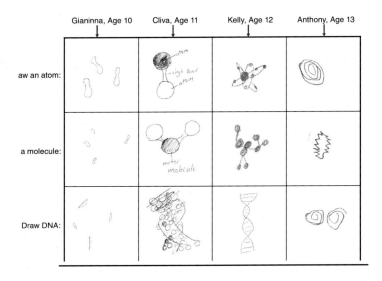

FIGURE 4-5 When asked to draw an atom, molecule, and piece of DNA, some children drew iconic ball-and-stick depictions of molecules and DNA (e.g., Cliva and Kelly), while others drew objects that bore no resemblance at all to how these materials are typically represented (e.g., Anthony).

SOURCE: Reprinted from Springer, *Journal of Nanoparticle Research,* Volume 10, Issue 7, 2008, pages 1141-1148, Numbers, scale and symbols: the public understanding of nanotechnology, CA Batt, AM Waldron, and N Broadwater, from Figure 3, Copyright © 2008, with kind permission from Springer Science and Business Media.

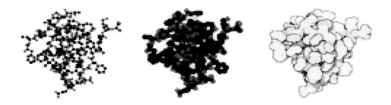

FIGURE 4-6 Interviewees were asked to identify components of each of these models of a molecule: ball-and-stick (on the left), space-filling (in the middle), and domain (on the right).

SOURCE: Reprinted from Springer, *Journal of Nanoparticle Research* Volume 10, Issue 7, 2008, pp 1141-1148, Numbers, scale and symbols: the public understanding of nanotechnology, CA Batt, AM Waldron, and N Broadwater, Copyright © 2008, with kind permission from Springer Science and Business Media. Reprinted with permission from David Goodsell, available online at http://www.rcsb.org/pdb/static.do?p=education_discussion/molecule_of_the_mo nth/pdb14_1.html. Accessed May 4, 2009.

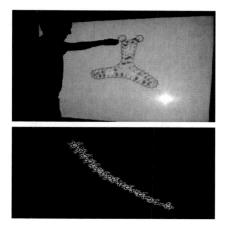

FIGURE 4-7 An exhibit in *Too Small to See* that was designed to communicate the concept that molecules are in constant motion. Visitors can reach out and fold and stretch the molecule on the screen.

Source: Reprinted with permission from Z. B. Simpson and Mine Control, Inc.; Reprinted with permission from A. Strickland.

Batt showed a picture of the exhibit when it was at Epcot Theme Park, Orlando, Florida, where 5,000 to 10,000 people toured the exhibition daily. He then showed some pictures of the various exhibits, including the following:

- *Magnification Station*, where visitors could see different size scales, including atomic scales (i.e., ball-and-stick molecular models), of some common objects, like an oyster shell, a butterfly wing and a salt crystal.
- *Zoom into Nation*, where visitors would turn a wheel to zoom in and out from the macroscopic to nanoscopic worlds. Batt said, "We had people just standing there for hours on end."
- *Build a Molecule*, where visitors would create their own molecular models. Batt said that kids would play at this station for 20–30 minutes at a time.
- *Atom Transporter*, where visitors would play an arcade-like game that involves arranging moving atoms into a pattern. Kids would spend abut 5–10 minutes at this station.

Batt and colleagues also built a smaller, bilingual version of the exhibit, *Too Small to See-2*, which is available for tour.

Nanooze and Other Nanotechnology Education Projects

Batt then briefly described *Nanooze*, which started as a webzine in 2006 (www.nanooze.org) and is now available in print as well. About 50,000 print copies of each issue are distributed across the United States. The webzine gets about 10,000 hits a month. The webzine is available in English, Spanish, Portuguese, and Swahili; it has primary articles, a blog, games, and interviews, and people can send questions, with a return time of about 90 minutes. Batt described *Nanooze* as "very cool" and pointed out that the last issue contains an interview with Don Eigler, a "gem of resources."

Batt also mentioned a partnership he and his group have with Earth-Sky (www.earthsky.org). Funded by the National Science Foundation (NSF); they are producing what they call "Chronicles of a Science Experiment," a series of 8-minute podcasts on nanotechnology and other science topics. In the first episode (September 8, 2008), Cornell University postdoctoral scientist Aaron Strickland talked about his daily life, not just in the lab but also at home. Batt said, "We're trying to give people this impression that science is back ... it actually involves pretty normal people ... pursuing interesting things."

In conclusion, Batt said that *Too Small to See* has been seen by about 5,000,000 visitors; *Nanooze* in print is seen by about 50,000 children, and *Nanooze* online gets about 10,000 hits a month; and EarthSky podcasts are heard 14 million times daily. He mentioned that the U.S. Department of Agriculture (USDA) would be sponsoring six EarthSky episodes on nanotechnology and food beginning in March 2009. A special issue of *Nanooze* will be produced to complement the podcasts.

CONSUMER INTEREST IN AND CONCERNS WITH EMERGING TECHNOLOGIES[8]

Presenter: Jean Halloran[9]

Scientific Knowledge Versus Acceptance of Technology

Halloran agreed with Moore and Batt that "consumers really don't know anything about nanotechnology," and she praised Batt's science education work, saying "If only it could be distributed everywhere because the sorry state of science education in a lot of the country is a real problem for the Nation." She expressed hope, however, that it wasn't being distributed with the expectation that, if people really understand nanotechnology, they will automatically accept its use in food. She emphasized that the two are "entirely separate questions." In fact, while not okay from an educational perspective, it may be okay from a "marketing perspective" if two-thirds of the public never really understand nanotechnology since they don't really need to learn about it unless it is causing some sort of problem. Consumers can become educated and tend to learn about new scientific entities or concepts very quickly when problems arise and something has them worried. For example, Halloran imagined that if people were polled two years ago about their knowledge of melamine, probably less than one percent of the population would have

---

[8] This section is a paraphrased summary of Jean Halloran's remarks. Unlike the other prepared presentations, Halloran shared thoughts and reactions to some of the key ideas and themes of the other presentations and discussions held throughout the day.
[9] Jean Halloran is Director of the Food Policies Initiative at the Consumers Union (publisher of *Consumer Reports*).

known what melamine was; today the majority of people probably know what melamine is.

Gaps in Scientific Knowledge About Safety

Halloran remarked that scientists involved with nanotechnology have been expressing a lot of enthusiasm about what they are doing with this new technology and where nanoscience is headed. This is an "absolutely natural thing for scientists to feel," she said. Unfortunately, however, we tend to hear only in passing that there are some safety issues. In fact, as Philbert stated, there is a huge gap in our scientific understanding of the safety of nanotechnology. For example, where exactly do nanoparticles go when they enter the human body?

Halloran suspects that grants are not being awarded for the scientific study of the safety of nanotechnology to nearly the same extent that they are being awarded for the investigation of "all the nifty new things you can do with nanotechnology." If such funding were available, Halloran said that scientists would probably be just as happy to address these safety questions. But now, without the funding, the attitude among nanoscientists is that addressing safety is not their job. They think it is someone else's responsibility.

Consumers' Fear of the Unknown

Halloran elaborated on a comment that Yada made during his overview presentation: that consumers fear the unknown. As a result of this fear of the unknown, one of the fastest-growing segments of the food market today is natural and organic food. Halloran said that this is not an unreasonable fear, for a couple of reasons. First, consumers tend to be conservative, or traditional, with foods. In other words, in scientific parlance, people have coevolved with their food supplies and without the benefit of what we can do with our food today because of science. People instinctively do things the "old way" or "the way that Grandma did things." People don't feel that innovation in food is really necessary. Second, consumers fear the unknown because of the way scientific innovations have been introduced over the past half-century. Consider, for example, synthetic chemicals: while they may do "incredible things" and have "probably brought us half the things in this room," they have also created all sorts of difficulties. We are in a situation now, for example, where we can't eat striped bass from the Hudson River because of poly-chlorinated biphenyl (PCB) contamination, and nobody knows how to fix the problem. The river itself has been cleaned, but cleaning the river bottom would cost billions and billions of dollars. So PCBs remain. Halloran pointed to the current debate about bisphenol A (BPA) as another example of the problems still emerging from our use of synthetic chemicals, with many people questioning how federal regulatory agencies are handling some of the issues.

Halloran argued that it is not "really fruitful" to have a discussion about whether consumers and the public are for or against nanotechnology. Rather, the issue is the safety and effectiveness of nanotechnology. The application of nanotechnology to the food supply needs to actually provide benefits to consumers and not be frivolous, and it needs to be safe. Of course, she said, there may be some consumers who would actually still appreciate having a "better Twinkie," so it may have some frivolous applications as well. Either way, it must be safe.

Regulating Nanotechnology in Food: Who Is Going to Do It and How?

This concern about safety raises the issue of regulation. Consumers want to know who is protecting them. Halloran remarked that, obviously, scientists are not going to ensure the safety of the applications they are developing, unless they receive the funding to do so. Nor, Halloran said, does FDA send a very reassuring message for consumers. She said, "It kind of feels like the FDA is sitting there waiting for the phone to ring." While some of the 800-plus products out there that are self-identified as "nano" may not even have nanoparticles in them, who is out there trying to figure out which ones do contain nanoparticles and, of those that do, whether they are safe? She agreed with Degnan's advice that written guidance needs to be provided so that at least sponsors know when they need to pick up the phone and call FDA. Halloran also noted that the Consumers Union, which she represents, has called for a mandatory safety review for the use of nanoparticles in all cosmetic and food products.

At this point, it falls on industry to ensure that products entering the market are safe, which raises another set of concerns. Experience has shown that industry has a difficult time regulating itself, even when it comes to its own long-term self-interest. There is such a premium on short-term gain that many products are pushed into the market without adequate self-assessment. Halloran argued that this is why FDA needs to be taking a more active role. Halloran referred to an earlier question (in the previous session) about companies that are developing products but for whom the cost of animal testing is prohibitive. So what are they doing? Are they moving forward with development anyway, without animal testing?

Consumer Choice

Halloran referred to the issue of choice that Moore brought up during her presentation. Consumers Union recognized the importance of this issue after some *Consumer Reports* testing with big commercial brand sunscreens revealed that the active ingredient in all sunscreens is either a chemical recognized by the Environmental Working Group as having some safety concerns or a nano-form of titanium dioxide or zinc oxide. A second round of testing with organic sunscreen products revealed that even though the customer service departments of these companies said that the products did not contain nanoparticles, in fact all of the products did. So there is no way at this point to avoid sunscreens with nanoparticles; the only other choice is to purchase a brand that contains a chemical recognized by the Environmental Working Group as being even more hazardous. The situation is exacerbated by the fact that the only reason nanoparticles are used in sunscreens is to make the lotions more transparent. Transparent sunscreens sell better than opaque ones, even though the benefit to consumers is not really that great. Halloran questioned whether consumers would really want transparent sunscreens if they really understood what was going on.

Other Safety Issues

Finally, Halloran referred to an earlier comment about vitamin fortification and asked whether it might be possible to get too much of a certain vitamin as a result of nanotechnology and, if so, how this could be prevented.

She identified the presence and use of nanoparticles in foods prepared in other countries and imported into the United States as another important but unresolved issue: Who is evaluating that? She noted the global nature of our food supply and that we are dealing with other countries that are just as technologically advanced as the United States but with weaker regulatory and safety infrastructures.

In conclusion, she advised, "go slow" and "be very, very precautionary to ensure it's safe."

PANEL DISCUSSION ON CURRENT ISSUES

All 10 speakers of the day were invited to participate as panelists during the final question and answer period. Much of the dialogue revolved around issues raised during this third session on consumer education and behavior, with Food Forum member Ned Groth's comments on consumer skepticism generating the most discussion. The issue of regulatory uncertainty was also revisited at length. More specifically, discussants considered:

- how consumers make new choices with new technologies;
- the lack of and need for more safety data on nanomaterials with novel properties and how regulatory guidance can be provided in the absence of such data;
- engaging the public in discussions about nanotechnology in food and empowering consumers;
- educating the public about nanotechnology;
- a comparison between consumer acceptance of nanotechnology in food and consumer acceptance of irradiation in food;
- naturally occurring food nanosystems and the positive spin they give to the concept of nanotechnology in food;
- second generation "nano-bio" devices being developed for the treatment of cancer and the regulatory challenges they will pose for the FDA;
- the various options FDA has for providing initial guidance on nanotechnologies in food;
- how other governments are dealing with these same issues; and
- how the United States will handle the importation of food products constructed with nanomaterials.

Consumer Choice and Demand

Doyle opened the panel discussion with a question about whether any research has been conducted to determine whether consumers would accept particular types of nanomaterials or approaches to nanotechnology in specific types of foods. Halloran replied first by stating that asking that type of question is oversimplified and would not provide a very useful response. If a product has been through a full safety review and the nanoscience/nanotechnology has been shown to provide some benefit that consumers could clearly identify, then yes, most consumers would almost certainly accept it. She remarked that some people draw an analogy with GMOs, but in fact nanotechnology doesn't raise the same "tampering with life" ethical issues. With nanotechnology, consumer acceptance is fundamentally a safety and usefulness matter.

Moore agreed with Halloran that consumers are more likely to respond to benefits than to risks. For example, there is a body of literature showing that the use of cell phones can promote brain tumors and cancers. Yet, most consumers view the benefits of cell phones as so great that the cell phone–brain tumor association will require a lot more evidence before people are willing to throw their cell phones away. She doesn't anticipate that type of response with nanotechnology in food. The public is still "up for grabs" with respect to being convinced of benefits associated with nanotechnology. She described some focus group work that the Project on Emerging Nanotechnologies has done with nano "toys," for example Tupperware that supposedly contains nano-silver particles with antimicrobial properties. When you put these "toys" in front of adults and ask them what they think, the overwhelming response is that people want more information—they want to know that the product is safe and who the authority figure is with respect to safety. But many people have a hard time identifying food safety authority figures that they trust. The authoritative source mentioned most often is *Consumer Reports*. She emphasized the necessity of having a food safety authority figure in place—it could be the Consumers Union (publisher of *Consumer Reports*), or it could be an FDA that people feel has been adequately resourced and provided with the tools necessary for overseeing safety. Taken together, research suggests that consumers are responsive to benefit, however, even in the absence of evidence for overwhelming benefit, consumers still need to be convinced by an authoritative figure before they will accept risks from a product.

Safety Data and Regulatory Guidance

Workshop attendee Scott Thurmond of the USDA remarked that there had been several calls during the course of the workshop for the FDA to promulgate guidance for nanomaterials to be submitted under their purview. The USDA is considering perhaps requesting absorption, distribution, metabolism, and excretion (ADME) data upfront for novel products, which Thurmond noted brings up another issue: while it easy to demand ADME data, it is much more difficult to demand how those data should be generated. He asked what advice the panel had for making that type of request. In response, Degnan suggested that rather than telling sponsors what they need to do, regulatory agencies could provide guidance in the form of questions (i.e., what type of questions the agency would ask when an actual petition for the product is submitted). That is just one suggestion, Degnan said, for dealing with "that type of knowledge vacuum." He remarked further that this is an area where regulatory authorities would benefit from the expertise of those people who have been studying and thinking about the applications of nanotechnology; such experts could help the regulatory agency determine the appropriate questions and identify issues that might arise, even before an actual product is under review.

Degnan again emphasized (as he had during his presentation) the value of having a written document to work with during those early stages, no matter how preliminary the guidance, particularly in cases where nanomaterials possessing novel properties have been added to products previously considered GRAS. With nanomaterials possessing novel properties, there is going to be a lot of focus on whether the GRAS exception is applicable or whether every additive with a nanomaterial with novel properties must go through the food additive approval process. "That, to me," he said, "is a really important regulatory issue that needs to be addressed in some manner."

Engaging the Public

Food Forum member Ned Groth made a couple of observations and said that he hoped his comments would stimulate some response from the panel. First, until he retired five years ago, he worked for 25 years for Consumers Union, where much of his work was in risk communication. During that time, he said, "I learned quite a bit about what consumers know and don't know and how they react to information." While consumers have a great deal of common sense, they also have enormous gaps in knowledge particularly with respect to quantitative information (as Batt elaborated during his presentation). For example, Consumers Union did some work with Alar about 20 years ago, when the pesticide was found in apple juice at parts per million (ppm) levels, exceeding EPA recommendations. When Consumers Union published that information, they received a lot of letters from concerned citizens, including a medical doctor from Rancho Cucamonga, California who asked what all the "fuss" was about, given that there "can't be more than one molecule" of Alar in a gallon of juice. In fact, at those ppm levels, a liter of apple juice would contain an astronomical number of molecules: 1.4×10^{17}. Groth said, "Even the people in this room probably couldn't get a good grip on it intellectually." Getting consumers to get a handle on this type of quantitative information is an enormous challenge.

The second observation Groth made was that, while consumers may not be very good with quantitative information, they are good with skepticism. He remarked that Yada's earlier comment about how the National Nanotechnology Initiative was designed to get kids excited about nanoscience and "all of the wonderful things that nanotechnology offers" reminded him of watching a Disney movie, *Our Friend the Atom*, as a kid, and then seeing 15–20 years later a pamphlet on nuclear power and electricity. The pamphlet, which was put out by a coalition of electrical utilities called Infinite Energy, claimed that nuclear power-generated electricity was going to be not only incredibly beneficial but also too cheap to meter and that the future would bring atomic cars, atomic airplanes, atomic wristwatches, etc. Then, 10–15 years later, there was an accident at Three Mile Island, and people realized that they had been hearing only part of the nuclear energy story. Generating this excitement serves a useful social purpose, Groth said, but consumers might wonder whether "sales pitches" like this are based on a balanced assessment of the public interest. Consumers are skeptical of both risks and benefits of new technologies. He referred to some of the data that Moore had presented which showed that many consumers think (without really knowing about the technology) that the risks are probably greater than the benefits or, at best, that the risks and benefits are the same. Groth argued that if participants in this stage of developing nanotechnology applications want to persuade consumers that there are in fact huge benefits to nanotechnology and not very big risks, they have to do it in a way that does not resemble a sales pitch. Instead, he encouraged efforts to engage consumers in the manner that Moore described: by inviting them to the table, finding out what they are interested in, including them in the decision-making process, and respecting their views (including their ignorance). This is very difficult and something, Groth said, "we haven't really learned to do very well as a society." He said that moving forward with nanotechnology "could be a big experiment in social mechanisms, as well as in new technology."

With respect to Groth's second observation (i.e., on public engagement), Moore agreed that the United States has not done a good job of engaging the public on science policy issues. Europe, she said, has done a "little better." In the United Kingdom, various government agencies have begun including interested citizens or consumers on oversight boards. One of the lessons learned in Europe is that unless people participate in a process and feel that their opinions and advice have some impact on the government decision-making, they feel like they are being given nothing more than a sales pitch and they become very angry. Moore expressed hope that, with new technology [i.e., not nanotechnology but new communication technology], society is developing "a new form of ... democracy." She stated that President Obama's use of the Internet while campaigning is a manifestation of this new type of democracy, one that entails a higher level of public engagement than has been possible in the past. She said that she doesn't think that these new avenues of communication have been explored enough as a way to truly engage the public and not just throw sales pitches.

Yada was the second panelist to comment on Groth's remarks. He commended the educational programming work that Batt is doing, but equally important will be conducting and communicating cost/benefit analyses. He remarked that the early stages of the GMO debate started with consumers stating that the technology was being imposed on them and without the public really understanding the technology.

Yada followed up with a question to Moore, asking if the data she presented on consumer perception of benefit/cost might be suspect if in fact only half of those surveyed actually understood the technology. He pointed out that if he were asked about the potential benefits and costs of a new technology that he did not understand, particularly with respect to that technology being applied in food, he wasn't sure that he could answer objectively. Moore confirmed that the one question pertaining to the benefits that people would like to see derived from nanotechnology was asked whether people knew about nanotechnology or not. She said its response was consistent with "virtually every finding" she is aware of with respect to the types of benefits people want from new technologies (i.e., that food and nutrition are not high priority benefits, and medical applications rank the highest). That finding is not nano-specific, she said.

Moore elaborated that, in fact, most consumers don't really make an effort to learn that much before making a decision, particularly a decision related to something scientific or technical. Sometimes they go to *Consumer Reports*, sometimes to a government or company website, but most of the time they turn to somebody they know who they consider reliable—it could be a cousin, a dentist or, for example when it comes to a cell phone, a 15-year-old boy. People turn to others who they think share the same values, are knowledgeable and accessible, and have your best interest in mind. Moore referred to a recent study reported in *Nature Nanotechnology*[10] concluding that most people form their attitudes and decisions about benefit/risk, for example whether nanotechnology is safe or unsafe, based on their "cultural cognition reality" and where they have "anchored" their trust. Once people have that cultural anchor, they process all other new pieces of data by turning to whomever it is they trust and processing their decisions accordingly. For example, people in some cultural groups mistrust industry declarations that products are safe because they don't think that industry has their best interest in mind. On the other hand, if you are in a different cultural group, for example if you are a 50-year-old white male businessperson, and GreenPeace declares that nanotechnology may be unsafe, you might automatically mistrust that declaration and believe that nanotechnology could provide a treatment for prostate cancer and that "those people don't want me to have it" or that "those people don't understand that we've got to make money in this country, that we've got to have a robust, technologically driven economy." Moore encouraged those who are trying to figure out how to engage the public in discussions about nanotechnology look at this research.

Philbert was the next to respond to Groth's comment by making an observation about some of the terms that people use when discussing nanotechnology. He said that while listening to this discussion, he keeps "bumping up against a simple cognitive dissonance and that is that we keep talking about this nanotechnology as if it's a thing." But it's not a single thing; nor is nanotoxicology. He also commented on use of the word "risk" and that there needs to be a careful distinction between "risk aversion" and "hazard aversion." Too often, when people use the word

---

[10] DM Kahan, D Braman, P Slovic, J Gastil, and G Cohen. 2008. Cultural cognition of the risks and benefits of nanotechnology. *Nature Nanotechnology* 4:87-94.

"risk," they are really referring to a "hazard." He also commented on the fact that as more is learned about nanotechnologies and their various applications, much of what has been learned to date will be supervened by new information. It is therefore very important that these discussions be open and transparent and that the public recognizes that "we're just lifting the edge of the rug." As we lift it further, much of the new information may very well reverse what will have already been said about the safety of nanomaterials up until that point. Nanotechnology is a very "sexy word," Philbert said, and a powerful inducer of grant funding, but it's useless for engaging the public and empowering consumers to make informed choices.

Moore agreed with Philbert "from an intellectual standpoint," but disagreed "from a practical standpoint." She said, "There are so many people who have embraced this word over the last 20-plus years in the vernacular, that I think its wishful thinking." She mentioned NSF awarding its first grant with nanotechnology in the title in 1991. She predicted that nanotechology would almost certainly be a major component of the Obama administration's economic stimulus package.

Philbert agreed with Moore on the widespread use of the word but opined that the language needs to evolve and that we need to go beyond using the simple "nanotechnology" label for everything nano. His fear, he said, is that something bad will eventually happen and that all useful nanotechnology, safe and otherwise, will be lost. Moore agreed.

Degnan responded next. Recognizing that biotechnology is "not the best comparator" for nanotechnology and that genetic alteration of natural materials raises a host of quite different concerns, there is a very clear practical lesson to be learned from that experience. Specifically, when biotechnology emerged, there was not single biotech product that consumers could identify with and recognize as being beneficial for them. Instead, the new technologies were benefiting the farmers, growers, and agricultural companies. After watching the biotech industry suffer injury for 15 years because of this, it is very clear that the first nanotechnology products that enter the market, whether they are medical care products or food packaging products (or something else), must possess recognizable consumer benefits.

Educating the Public About Nanotechnology

Food Forum member Donna Porter, who also served on the workshop planning committee, asked the panelists a series of questions, beginning with two questions directed at Batt. First, have Batt and his colleagues been able to test people's knowledge after they have been through *Too Small to See*? Second, is there any plan to expand the exhibition into, for example, a school program that could be presented by teachers nationwide? Batt said the answer to both questions was "yes." Regarding the first, because the exhibit receives NSF support, some sort of assessment is required, so he and his team have in fact done that. He referred workshop attendees to www.informalscience.org for a summary of what Batt and his team have learned about what people gain from the exhibit. Regarding the second question, the exhibit is currently on national tour. It rotates from one science museum to the next about every three months. Its touring schedule is posted online at www.toosmall tosee.org.

Nanoooze is being distributed nationwide as well. It is being sent mostly to teachers, although anybody can request copies. The big challenge, Batt said, is that every state has their own formal education agenda/curriculum and not a single one of those curricula include nanotechnology. He said, "To try to shove that into the curriculum as a mandate is virtually impossible." He and his team are doing what they can to distribute *Nanooze* as much as possible. Porter asked if it has been presented at science teacher education conferences. Batt said yes, for example the National Science Teachers Association (NSTA). He mentioned that after *Nanooze* was recently reviewed in a newsletter, *Neuroscience for Kids*, Batt asked the newsletter editor where he had heard about *Nanooze* and learned that it was being distributed among various language arts programs as well. Batt said that it's very graphically pleasing, with a lot of "cool stuff," and it is not just being read in the science classroom.

Comparing Consumer Acceptance of Nanotechnology to Consumer Acceptance of Irradiation

Porter then directed two questions to Moore and Philbert. First, has the consumer reaction to nanotechnology been similar to what occurred when irradiation in food was first discussed? Second, when new technological ideas are presented to consumers, for example in focus groups or through polling studies, are consumers led to believe that all food is going to be affected by the new technology (whether it be irradiation or, today, nanotechnology), or do the respondents understand that the new technologies will be used only in selected ways, at least initially? Moore said that, based on four years of focus group work, her informed opinion is that people generally react to nanotechnology as being something "cool." It sounds "hip and edgy," particularly to the younger generation. But there is not a lot of awareness about what nanotechnology is. In the first focus group she conducted (four years ago), when asked if anybody had ever heard about nanotechnology, only a few participants responded, and somewhat tentatively. In the last series of focus groups, conducted in August 2008, 10 of 12 pairs of hands shot up when the same question was asked. However, when further asked how they had heard about it, many people mentioned the iPod nano. But, Porter said, "at least they got that it was small. They got the first 'Carl Commandment' down." So awareness of nanotechology remains the same (i.e., low).

The reaction to synthetic biology, Moore said, has been more similar to what occurred with irradiated food. The word "synthetic" brings to mind nylon and other images of things that were "new and great and wonderful" decades ago but are not thought of that way today. Today, consumers want things that are "organic" and "natural." When "synthetic" is combined with "biology," people who know even less about synthetic biology than they know about nanotechnology don't like it. There is a "yuck factor" associated with synthetic biology, as there was with irradiated food, that many people "are just not going to get over." Use of the word "nanotechnology" does not elicit that same response. Just with the nomenclature, she said "you're starting off at a better point than you might think you are."

Halloran agreed that nanotechnology is starting out with a "good rap" and that the iPod nano had done the technology a "huge favor." Irradiation in food, on the other hand, started out as being associated with an effect of the atomic bomb and, as such, had to cross a huge hurdle. Either way, the public does not get enough credit for the "reasonable and rational way" they make their back-of-the-envelope risk/benefit analyses. With irradiated food, public perception was also influenced, for example, by a *Consumer Reports* project on irradiated food showing that irradiated meat did taste differently, that the irradiation did not kill all bacteria and potentially created a false sense of security, and that there were other ways to make meat safer. That was how *Consumer Reports* came to their conclusion about irradiated meat (i.e., not by associating it with effects of the atomic bomb), and that is how the average consumer forms his or her opinion as well. Halloran remarked further that not only do these technologies (irradiation and nanotechnology) involve complex decisions, those decisions are often made within the context of individual applications and on a case-by-case basis. This is particularly true of the use of nanotechnology in food. Not only does each nanotechnology have different benefits, those benefits depend on the (food structure) matrix and all of the other variables that must be taken into consideration when conducting safety analyses. We can't make broad generalizations about whether nanotechnology is good or bad.

Naturally Occurring Nanosystems

Food Forum member Eric Decker interjected with a comment on the common perception that processed foods are "evil" and that the addition of synthetic nanotechnology-derived compounds to foods would make consumers even more wary of processed foods. Yet, as Aguilera discussed during his presentation, many nanostructures naturally exist in foods. Not only do we consume nanostructures all the time, but also these nanostructures are often what make foods "good for us." Casein micelles, which deliver calcium, are just one example. Decker stated that there has not been enough scientific exploration of naturally occurring nanosystems and the benefits they provide and that conducting more of that type of analysis would provide the means for telling a very positive story about a technology that "could be beneficial to everybody."

The Use of Nanotechnology to Treat Cancer

Recognizing that the question was slightly off-topic, Porter then asked Philbert about the current status of using nanotechnology to treat cancer. Philbert said, "It is here." There are at least two nanotechnology-derived formulations for anticancer therapeutics that are already FDA approved. Both are smaller reformulations of existing drugs. There is also a second wave of nanoscale approaches being applied in medicine where "nano" is no longer the "watchword" and where FDA "is going to hit the wall." Philbert described these second-wave approaches as "nano-bio." He and his colleagues, for example, are working on nano-bio hybrids of polymers and bioactive peptides for use in drug and contrast agent delivery. Philbert predicted that the FDA will not only have a difficult time categorizing some of these second-wave products, which fall somewhere between drugs and devices, but the agency will also have a difficult time evaluating their safety. It is very difficult to predict how the various components of many of these products break down.

The Starting Point for Regulatory Guidance

The focus of the discussion shifted back to issues related to safety and regulatory guidance when Porter asked Degnan and Tarantino if the FDA would be providing initial guidance with an Advanced Notice of Proposed Rulemaking (ANPR), commenting that this is how many other issues without proposed rules were started. Degnan replied that an ANPR is more time-consuming than guidance. If the guidance is structured as preliminary but thought-provoking, it could serve the same purpose as an ANPR with respect to "attracting attention, scrutiny, comment, and a level of thoughtfulness and attention that at least I haven't seen to date."

Tarantino agreed. She said that guidance makes more sense than an ANPR if for no other reason than it is easier to change than a regulation, at least at this point. She referred to Degnan's earlier comments about the importance of including questions about safety in the initial guidance and suggested that some of the questions asked at the public meeting on September 8, 2008, might serve as a good starting point. If a regulation in a certain area were to become useful, however, an ANPR would be a good way to solicit maximum input and ensure transparency. The goal, Tarantino said, is to encourage as much dialogue and involvement as possible.

Degnan followed up by remarking that FDA in fact has a number of options and that multiple routes could be taken. Historically, FDA has simply used notices in the Federal Register to post questions. In the late 1980s, for example, prior to passage of the Nutrition Labeling and Education Act (NLEA), FDA issued a number of questions about how to regulate nutrition (e.g., whether mandatory nutrition is necessary and what authority FDA would have). As another example, about five or six years ago, FDA issued a similar notice asking questions about over-the-counter (OTC) drugs (e.g., Is this an appropriate way to proceed?). Finally, just a couple of months ago (in July/August 2008), FDA issued a notice in the Federal Register asking questions about the newly enacted section 912 of the FDC Act. So rather than taking a position one way or the other, the agency asks some "very probing questions." Publishing a notice of this nature would be another way to initiate dialogue.

How Other Governments Are Dealing with
Nanotechnology Regulation

Porter asked Yada and Aguilera how their governments were proceeding with nanotechnology regulation in food. Aguilera said that the Chilean government is only just beginning to talk about nanotechnology and that there is no specific initiative dealing with nanotechnology applications in food. It will become an important issue in the near future, however, since Chile exports more foods than most other Latin American countries. Yada replied that the situation in Canada is similar to that of the United States, with regulatory authorities still struggling with the issue. Many questions are being debated: Are we going to regulate the technology? Are we going to regulate the products? What guidelines will we use? Will we use the precautionary principle? Will we use substantial equivalencies? Yada noted that he had recently visited Ottawa, where he consulted with Canadian food inspection agency regulators who were "really probing" to identify the issues needing attention.

Finally, Porter asked the other panelists if they knew of any other government that has moved ahead with respect to regulation of food nanotechnology. Halloran commented that the European Union (EU) had requested information on sunscreens with nanomaterials, which Halloran interpreted as an encouraging sign. More specifically, the EU requested that manufacturers provide safety data within a year (of the request). Wolf Maier of the EU commented that the UK Parliament was considering a motion to regulate all foods that contain particles derived from nanotechnology as normal foods, which would mean that they are subject to pre-market authorization. While the issue is not yet decided, the questioner remarked that pre-market authorization seems to be the direction headed.

Tarantino offered a final remark: The EU food safety authority had issued a call for data and information to aid in its review process and also was receiving expert advice from the World Health Organization (WHO) and Food and Agriculture Organization (FAO). So agencies worldwide are gathering information in an effort to decide how best to proceed.

Importing Food Products That Contain Nanomaterials

Doyle noted that the first four speakers of the day were from outside of the United States and that obviously there is a lot of international activity in the area of food nanotechnology. He asked, how will the United States address the import of nanotechnology-derived foods? Degnan responded by stating that FDA's authority over imports is its broadest authority and that the agency can detain a product based simply on the appearance of a violation. It is a very tough standard—appearing to be a violation is very different than having been proven to be a violation. But the FDA needs to be prepared, he said, so that regulatory decisions are not being made in an enforcement context. Regulatory decisions need to be made in a deliberate, meaningful, structured way with respect to both statutory standards and available science.

Tarantino said that the easy answer is that all imported foods must meet U.S. safety standards, "whatever those are." The bigger issue is how do you do that? She agreed with Degnan that the FDA needs to be prepared. She said, "I think trying to stay abreast of what actually is happening not only in this country but elsewhere is, right now, the best we can do to … anticipate what we are likely to be seeing." The workshop was then adjourned.

A

Workshop Agenda

**Nanotechnology in Food Products:
Impact on Food Science, Nutrition and the Consumer**

The National Academies Keck Center
Room 100
500 Fifth Street, NW
Washington, DC

December 10, 2008

**8:00–
8:30 am** **Registration**

INTRODUCTION

8:30 am **Welcome from Food Forum**
Mike Doyle, Chair of the Food Forum

8:40 am **Opening Remarks
Nanotechnology: A New Frontier in Foods, Food
Packaging, and Nutrient Delivery**
Rickey Yada, University of Guelph

SESSION 1: APPLICATION OF NANOTECHNOLOGY TO FOOD PRODUCTS

9:00 am **Overview of Nanosciences and Food**
*José Miguel Aguilera, Universidad Católica de Chile,
Santiago*

9:20 am **Application of Nanotechnology in Rapid Detection of
Food Pathogens**
Frans Kampers, Wageningen University

9:40 am   **Use of Nanomaterials to Improve Food Quality and**
                   Food Safety: Nutrient Encapsulation and Food
                   Packaging
                   Jochen Weiss, University of Hohenheim, Stuttgart

10:00 am   **Questions and Discussion**

10:30 am   **BREAK**

SESSION 2: SAFETY AND EFFICACY OF NANOMATERIALS IN FOOD PRODUCTS

11:00 am   **A Biological Perspective on Nanostructures in Foods**
                   Martin Philbert, University of Michigan, Ann Arbor

11:20 am   **FDA Oversight of Nanotechnology Applications in**
                   Foods, Food Packaging, and Nutrient Delivery
                   Laura Tarantino, Food and Drug Administration

11:40 am   **Regulatory Issues Concerning Food and**
                   Nutrient Products Containing Nanomaterials
                   Fred Degnan, King and Spaulding

12:00 pm   **Questions and Discussion**

12:30–
1:30 pm   **LUNCH**

SESSION 3: EDUCATING AND INFORMING CONSUMERS ABOUT APPLICATIONS OF NANOTECHNOLOGY TO FOOD PRODUCTS

1:30 pm   **Nanotechnology and Food: The Public Knows**
                   "Nano"
                   Julia Moore, Woodrow Wilson International Center for
                   Scholars

1:50 pm   **Challenges in Educating Consumers About Emerging Technologies**
Carl Batt, Cornell University

2:10 pm   **Discussion: Consumer Interest in and Concerns with Emerging Technologies**
Jean Halloran, Consumers Union

2:30 pm   **Panel Discussion on Current Issues**
All Speakers

3:30 pm   **Adjourn**

B

Workshop Participants

Diaa Ahmed
Utrecht University
Arlington, VA

Norri Alderson
FDA
Rockville, MD

Sue Anne Assimon
FDA
College Park, MD

Jeffrey Barach
GAO
Washington, DC

Geoffrey Becker
Library of Congress
Washington, DC

Samuel Besong
Delaware State University
Dover, DE

Kristie Bowman
U.S. Pharmacopeia
Rockville, MD

Richard Bruner
WIL/Biotechnics, LLC
Clemson, SC

Betty Bugusu
IFT
Washington, DC

Robert Bursey
Ajinomoto Corporate Services
   LLC
Washington, DC

Jean Buzby
USDA
Washington, DC

Tim Callahan
Organic Trade Association
Greenfield, MA

Elizabeth Calvey
FDA
College Park, MD

Richard Canady
FDA
Rockville, MD

Chris Cannizzaro
U.S. State Department
Washington, DC

Ricardo Carvajal
Hyman, Phelps, & McNamara,
  P.C.
Washington, DC

Kimberly Cassidy
FDA
College Park, MD

Velma Charles-Shannon
USDA
Washington, DC

Robert Collette
Institute of Shortening and
  Edible Oils
Washington, DC

Paul Cotton
NIH
Bethesda, MD

Rebecca Danam
FDA
College Park, MD

Cindy Davis
NCI
Rockville, MD

Kerry Dearfield
USDA
Washington, DC

Katya Delak
U.S. Department of State
Washington, DC

Sarah Delea
Kraft Foods
Northfield, IL

Darinka Djordjevic
ILSI North America
Washington, DC

Scott Douglas
HHS
Washington, DC

Michael Doyle
University of Georgia
Griffin, GA

Laura Dye
FDA
College Park, MD

Paul Earhart
K Consulting
Alexandria, VA

Katie Egan
FDA
College Park, MD

Jessica Eisner
U.S. Department of State
Washington, DC

Leland Ellis
Department of Homeland
  Security
Washington, DC

Kathleen, Ellwood
FDA
College Park, MD

Nancy Emenaker
NCI
Rockville, MD

Abby Ershow
NIH
Bethesda, MD

Bianca Farias
FDA
College Park, MD

Brian Ferrar
British Embassy
Washington, DC

Eric Flamm
FDA
Rockville, MD

Vasiliki Flari
FDA
College Park, MD

Sabine Francke-Carroll
FDA
College Park, MD

Steve Froggett
USDA
Washington, DC

Thomas Fungwe
USDA
Alexandria, VA

Eric Garber
FDA
College Park, MD

Matthew Gerdin
U.S. Department of State
Washington, DC

Marietta Gubuan
Washington, DC

Bill Gulledge
American Chemistry Council
Arlington, VA

Kiros Hailemariam
FDA
College Park, MD

Brenda Halbrook
USDA
Alexandria, VA

Diane Hannemann
U.S. Department of State
Washington, DC

Gail Hansen
U.S. Senate
Washington, DC

Darlene Hardie-Muncy
Cargill
Wayzata, MN

Moti Harel
Advanced Bionutrition Corp
Columbia, MD

Molly Harry
FDA
College Park, MD

David Hattan
FDA
College Park, MD

Valerie Hernandez-Hansen
LRRI
Springfield, VA

Jane Ho
USDA
Washington, DC

Terrance Horner
GAO
Washington, DC

Yvonne Jackson
Administration on Aging
Washington, DC

Gregory Jaffe
CSPI
Washington, DC

Gita Jayan
FDA
Rockville, MD

William Jordan
EPA
Washington, DC

Emi Kameyama
The National Academies
Washington, DC

Mark Kantor
University of Maryland
College Park, MD

Lisa Katic
K Consulting
Alexandria, VA

David Kelly
FDA
Rockville, MD

Abu Khan
FDA
College Park, MD

Henry Kim
FDA
College Park, MD

Antony Klapper
Reed Smith, LLP
Washington, DC

Kathleen Koehler
HHS
Washington, DC

Todd Kuiken
Woodrow Wilson International
    Center for Scholars
Washington, DC

Rachel Lange
FDA
College Park, MD

Angela Lasher
FDA
College Park, MD

Rachel Lattimore
Arent Fox, LLP
Washington, DC

Hyoung Lee
FDA
College Park, MD

Joseph A. Levitt
Hogan & Hartson, LLP
Washington, DC

James Lindsay
USDA
Beltsville, MD

Arthur Lipman
FDA
College Park, MD

Markus Lipp
US Pharmacopeia
Rockville, MD

Ronald Lorentzen
FDA
College Park, MD

Kerri Lowrey
The MayaTech Corporation
Silver Spring, MD

Hnin Yu Lwin
Brandeis University
Alexandria, VA

Douglas MacKay
Council for Responsible
  Nutrition
Washington, DC

Patricia MacNeil
USDA
Alexandria, VA

Wolf Maier
European Commission
  Delegation
Washington, DC

Subhas Malghan
FDA
Silver Spring, MD

Andrew Mara
National Defense University
Washington, DC

Robert Martin
FDA
College Park, MD

Crystal McDade-Ngutter
NIH
Bethesda, MD

Carrie McMahon
FDA
College Park, MD

Jianghong Meng
University of Maryland
College Park, MD

Christine Micheel
Institute of Medicine
Washington, DC

Jeremy Mihalov
FDA
College Park, MD

Nancy Miller
NIH
Bethesda, MD

John Milner
NCI
Rockville, MD

Dragan Momcilovic
FDA
Rockville, MD

Sylvester Mosley
FDA
College Park, MD

Clarence Murray
FDA
College Park, MD

Mary Nucci
Food Policy Institute
New Brunswick, NJ

Susan Offutt
GAO
Washington, DC

Mickey Parish
University of Maryland
College Park, MD

Robin Parsell
Institute of Medicine
Washington, DC

Cheryl Pellerin
U.S. Department of State
Washington, DC

Andrew Perraut
OMB
Washington, DC

Donna Porter
Library of Congress
Washington, DC

Lauren Posnick Robin
FDA
College Park, MD

Edward Puro
FDA
College Park, MD

P. Isaac Rabbani
FDA
College Park, MD

Moraima Ramos Valle
FDA
College Park, MD

Ram Rao
USDA
Washington, DC

Jim Rasekh
USDA
Washington, DC

Penelope Rice
FDA
College Park, MD

Steven Rizk
Mars Incorporated
Hackettstown, NJ

Sharon Ross
NCI
Bethesda, MD

Annette Santamaria
ENVIRON
Houston, TX

John Sargent
Library of Congress
Washington, DC

Morton Satin
Salt Institute
Rockville, MD

Betty Shackleford
EPA
Arlington, VA

Lisa Shames
GAO
Washington, DC

Tyler Shannon
Food & Water Watch
Washington, DC

Kaniz Shireen
FDA
College Park, MD

Linda Singletary
USDA
Washington, DC

Isabelle Slight
Health Canada
Ottawa, Ontario, Canada

Jennifer Smith
FDA
Arlington, VA

Pothur Srinivas
NIH
Bethesda, MD

Jannavi Srinivasan
FDA
College Park, MD

Pamela Starke-Reed
NIH
Bethesda, MD

Stephen Sundlof
FDA
College Park, MD

Shirley Tao
FDA
College Park, MD

Scott Thurmond
FDA
College Park, MD

Mary Torrence
USDA
Beltsville, MD

Nga Tran
Exponent
Washington, DC

Elaine Trujillo
NCI
Bethesda, MD

Sylvia Trujillo
American Medical Association
Washington, DC

Saleh Turujman
FDA
College Park, MD

Robert Vimini
Perdue Farms
Salisbury, MD

Qin Wang
University of Maryland
College Park, MD

Lisa Watson
Watson/Mulhern
Washington, DC

Jennifer Weber
ADA
Washington, DC

Elizabeth Williams
University of Maryland
Bethesda, MD

Samuel Williams
Southern Christian Leadership
Frederick, MD

Robert Winters
Hogan & Hartson
Washington, DC

Violet Woo
NIH
Bethesda, MD

Sibyl Wright
USDA
Washington, DC

Wenying Wu
Smithsonian Institution
Washington, DC

Vladimir Yurovsky
FDA
College Park, MD

C

Speaker Biographies

José Miguel Aguilera, Ph.D., is Professor of Food Engineering at the P. Universidad Católica de Chile in Santiago. He has contributed to food technology and engineering, specifically the study of food microstructure, undertaking research in areas such as structure-property relationships in foods and biomaterials; applications of modern microscopy techniques; and modeling and quantitation of microstructural changes in foods. Dr. Aguilera is associate editor of the Journal of Food Science and is a member of the editorial board of Food Biophysics and Trends in Food Science & Technology, among others. He also serves as a consultant to the Nestlé Research Center and to Unilever.

Carl A. Batt, Ph.D., is Liberty Hyde Bailey Professor of Food Science and codirector of the Nanobiotechnology Center (NBTC), and Director of the Cornell University/Ludwig Institute for Cancer Research Partnership. He is cofounder and former director of the Nanobiotechnology Center and serves as the faculty mentor for all Public Service Center educational programs, which span from pre-K through graduate education. In collaboration with community partners, Dr. Batt has established science clubs in three rural middle schools that are focused on getting young women excited about science, and is the founder of the webzine, *Nanooze*, that is distributed throughout the United States and translated into three other languages.

Fred H. Degnan, joined King & Spalding's food and drug practice in 1988 after an 11-year career in the Food and Drug Administration's Office of General Counsel. Since 1989 he has taught food and drug law at the Catholic University of America where he serves as a Distinguished Lecturer. He has numerous publications including the book *FDA's*

Creative Application of the Law (2d ed., 2006). While at FDA he received the agency's highest awards and in 2002 received the FDLI Distinguished Leadership award. He has consistently been recognized in numerous independently conducted surveys as being among the nation's top food and drug lawyers.

Michael Doyle, Ph.D., is Regents Professor of Food Microbiology and director of the University of Georgia Center for Food Safety. His research focuses on developing methods to detect and control foodborne bacterial pathogens at all levels of the food continuum, from the farm to the table. He is internationally acknowledged as a leading authority on foodborne pathogens.

Jean Halloran is Director of Food Policy Initiatives at Consumers Union, publisher of *Consumer Reports*. Ms. Halloran is responsible for developing policy and staff initiatives on biotechnology, mad cow disease prevention, mercury in fish, and meat and produce contamination. She presently serves on the U.S. State Department's Advisory Committee on International Economic Policy, and formerly served on the National Academy of Sciences' Board on Agriculture and Natural Resources. Ms. Halloran helped organize the Trans Atlantic Consumer Dialogue (TACD), a coalition of groups in Europe and the United States and serves as its U.S. liaison point. She represented Consumers International at Codex Alimentarius in negotiations that developed standards for safety assessment of genetically engineered foods.

Frans Kampers, Ph.D., is co-coordinator of research on nanotechnology in food at Wageningen UR, The Netherlands. He is also director of BioNT, the virtual centre for bio-nanotechnology in Wageningen. He is one of the initiators of the Nano4Food conference and is actively involved in the organization of new funding programs in The Netherlands. Dr. Kampers is a former member of the Dutch agricultural research organization where he was department head and investigative leader of instrumentation and measurement technology. He is frequently interviewed and invited to speak on the subject of nanotechnology in food.

Julia Moore is Deputy Director of the Project on Emerging Nanotechnologies, a joint initiative of the Woodrow Wilson International Center for Scholars and The Pew Charitable Trusts. The project is designed to help businesses, governments, and the public anticipate and manage the possible health and environmental implications of nanotechnology. Formerly, she was Senior Advisor in the Office of International Science and Engineering at the National Science Foundation (NSF) and she was Director of Legislative & Public Affairs at NSF.

Martin A. Philbert, Ph.D., is Professor of Environmental Sciences, and Senior Associate Dean for Research at the University of Michigan, School of Public Health. Dr. Philbert's research interests include the development of nanotechnology for intracellular measurement of biochemicals and ions, and for the early detection and treatment of brain tumors. He is the recipient of the 2001 Society of Toxicology Achievement Award. Dr. Philbert provides consultation to the National Cancer Institute, National Institute of Environmental Health Sciences, the National Toxicology Program, and is a scientific advisor to the International Life Sciences Institute in Washington, DC.

Laura Tarantino, Ph.D., is Director of the Office of Food Additive Safety in the Center for Food Safety and Applied Nutrition, U.S. Food and Drug Administration. The Office of Food Additive Safety is responsible for managing the safety evaluation of substances added to food, including food and color additives and substances that are Generally Recognized as Safe (GRAS) as well as of new plant varieties developed using recombinant DNA methods. Dr. Tarantino has been involved in the development and implementation of regulatory policies pertaining to food and color additives and GRAS ingredients, food irradiation, and new food varieties developed using methods of modern biotechnology.

Jochen Weiss, Ph.D., is Professor of Food Science at the University of Hohenheim in Germany. His current research interest is in the area of fabrication of novel colloidal and nanostructures that can be used as encapsulation or delivery systems of functional food ingredients. In addition, he investigates the application of high-intensity ultrasound for use in food structuring and processing. Dr. Weiss is the recipient of the 2007 Institute of Food Technologists Young Scientist Samuel L. Prescott Award.

Rickey Yada, Ph.D., is Professor in the Department of Food Science and a Canada Research Chair in Food Protein Structure at the University of Guelph. He is also Scientific Director of the Advanced Foods and Materials Network within the Networks of Centres of Excellence Program (NCE) of Canada. His primary research focus is structure-dynamics-function relations of food-related proteins. Dr. Yada is a Fellow of the Canadian Institute of Food Science and Technology and of the International Academy, International Union of Food Science and Technology and was a member of the Royal Society of Canada Expert Panel on the Future of Food Biotechnology.

D

Acronyms and Abbreviations

ADME	absorption, distribution, metabolism, and excretion
Ag	silver
ANPR	Advanced Notice of Proposed Rulemaking
BPA	bisphenol A
CIIT	Chemistry Industry Institute of Toxicology
CN	carbon nanotube
CSREES	Cooperative State Research, Education, and Extension Service (a USDA agency)
DNRC	Division of Nutrition Research Service Coordination (an NIH agency)
EPA	Environmental Protection Agency
EU	European Union
FAA	Food Additives Amendment
FAO	Food and Agriculture Organization
FDA	Food and Drug Administration
FDC	Food, Drug, and Cosmetic
GFP	green fluorescent protein
GI	gastrointestinal
GLP	Good Laboratory Practice
GMA	Grocery Manufacturers Association
GMO	genetically modified organism

GRAS	Generally Recognized as Safe
HHP	high hydrostatic pressure
IFBC	International Food Biotechnology Council
IFT	Institute of Food Technologists
IOM	Institute of Medicine
NDI	New Dietary Ingredients
NIEHS	National Institute of Environmental Health Sciences
NIH	National Institutes of Health
nm	nanometer
NLEA	Nutrition Labeling and Education Act
NNI	National Nanotechnology Initiative
NSET	Nanoscale Science, Engineering, and Technology (a subcommittee of the NNI)
NSF	National Science Foundation
NSTA	National Science Teachers Association
OSHA	Occupational Safety and Health Administration
OTC	over-the-counter
PCB	polychlorinated biphenyl
RFID	radio frequency identification device
SLN	solid lipid nanoparticle
SWCNT	single-walled carbon nanotube
UBC	University of British Columbia
USDA	U.S. Department of Agriculture
WHO	World Health Organization